Steven Hoyanowsky
1608 Mc Pherson Blvd.
Fremont, Ohio 43420

Coronary Care Nursing

SHEILA H. HUANG, R.N., M.S.

Assistant Manager, Education and
   Training Department
Northwest Hospital, Seattle, Washington

LYNNE A. DASHER, R.N., B.S.N., C.C.R.N.

Staff Nurse, Critical Care Unit
Northwest Hospital, Seattle, Washington
Cardiac Nurse Consultant for Holter
   Scanning Division of Pathologist
   Central Laboratory, Seattle, Washington

**CHRISTINE ASHLEY LARSON,
R.N., M.N., C.C.R.N.**

Instructor, School of Health Sciences
Seattle Pacific University

**CAROLYN D. McCULLOCH,
R.N., M.N., C.C.R.N.**

Staff Nurse, Critical Care Unit
Northwest Hospital, Seattle, Washington

1983
W. B. SAUNDERS COMPANY
Philadelphia   London   Toronto
Mexico City   Rio de Janeiro   Sydney   Tokyo

W. B. Saunders Company: West Washington Square
Philadelphia, PA 19105

1 St. Anne's Road
Eastbourne, East Sussex BN21 3UN, England

1 Goldthorne Avenue
Toronto, Ontario M8Z 5T9, Canada

Apartado 26370—Cedro 512
Mexico 4, D.F., Mexico

Rua Coronel Cabrita, 8
Sao Cristovao Caixa Postal 21176
Rio de Janeiro, Brazil

9 Waltham Street
Artarmon, N.S.W. 2064, Australia

Ichibancho, Central Bldg., 22-1 Ichibancho
Chiyoda-Ku, Tokyo 102, Japan

Library of Congress Cataloging in Publication Data

Main entry under title:

Coronary care nursing.

1. Cardiovascular disease nursing.   I. Huang, Sheila H.

RC674.C69 1983   616.1'2'0024613   82–42507

ISBN 0–7216–4799–5

Coronary Care Nursing   ISBN   0-7216-4799-5

Last digit is the print number: 9   8   7   6   5   4   3   2   1

INTRODUCTORY NOTE

The Saunders Blue Books Series is intended to provide, in a handy, convenient format, up-to-date information about therapy and patient care across a wide range of clinical fields. Blue Books are designed to help practicing physicians, nurses, emergency personnel, and other health care professionals and students to deliver quality patient care. Our series derives its title from the very first W. B. Saunders publication (Hare: *Essentials of Physiology*, Saunders, 1888). This book was part of a famous list of 24-question compends known as the "Blue Series." The purpose of that series was to sort out important scientific and clinical facts so that students could review and assess their knowledge. The name of the present series reflects its heritage from that pioneering venture. Today, when scientific information is growing exponentially, health professionals recognize an increasing obligation both to remain current and to select from this sea of facts those that add significantly to that foundation upon which sound clinical practice is based. The Blue Books address this need. They should not be regarded as textbooks or office references, but as portable clinical tools—as vital to quality patient care as a stethoscope or blood pressure cuff.

MICKEY S. EISENBERG, M.D., PH.D.
Consulting Editor, Blue Books Series

PREFACE

Because of the ever-changing conditions of coronary patients, nurses caring for these patients are required to make precise and timely decisions. The purpose of this book is to provide essential information needed for decision-making and for appropriate nursing interventions in an easily followed format with clear titles and subtitles. The content encompasses cardiac disorders commonly seen in Coronary Care Units. It is not intended for a comprehensive, in-depth coverage of coronary care nursing. However, the scope of the book is sufficiently broad to serve as a quick reference in the clinical area and as a guide for self-learning in coronary care nursing.

SHEILA H. HUANG
LYNNE A. DASHER
CHRISTINE ASHLEY LARSON
CAROLYN D. McCULLOCH

ACKNOWLEDGMENTS

The authors wish to thank Dr. Mickey Eisenberg and Miss Katherine Pitcoff for their continuous advice and support throughout the development of the manuscript and our family members for their encouragement and accommodation of family schedule changes.

We express our appreciation for the fine work done by our illustrator, Mr. Ivan Buck, and the typist, Miss Karen Sheide.

Special thanks are also due to Charlotte Varner for her initial organization of the writing team and to Mrs. Laurel Beresford, Dr. John Murray, Mr. Ken Hall and Miss Marilyn Carlson for their various assistance.

CONTENTS

Coronary Atherosclerosis

Angina Pectoris

Myocardial Infarction

Sudden Cardiac Death

Chapter 12

Sinus Rhythms

Atrial Rhythms

Junctional Rhythms (AV Nodal Rhythms)

Ventricular Rhythms

Atrioventricular Block

Intraventricular Conduction Defects

Pre-Excitation Syndrome

Chapter 13

CONGESTIVE HEART FAILURE 204

Chapter 14

SHOCK.. 216

Chapter 15

HYPERTENSION 229

Chapter 16

MISCELLANEOUS DISORDERS 244

Pericarditis and Cardiac Tamponade

Pericarditis

Cardiac Tamponade

Myocarditis

Infective Endocarditis

Rheumatic Heart Disease

Cardiomyopathy

Idiopathic Hypertrophic Subaortic Stenosis (IHSS)

Cor Pulmonale

Section IV   SPECIFIC MEDICAL THERAPIES

Chapter 17

MEDICATIONS COMMONLY USED IN CCU........ 284

Section V CARDIAC REHABILITATION

Section VI APPENDICES

NURSING ASSESSMENT

1

NURSING ASSESSMENT OF THE CARDIAC PATIENT

GENERAL CONSIDERATIONS

It is through assessment that the nurse determines the needs of the patient, thus enabling appropriate nursing interventions. Assessment comprises two basic components: observation (including general appearance and behavior, auscultation, palpation, and percussion) and communication (including interview and nursing history).

The gathering of this data is facilitated by helping the patient to understand the value and use of the information to be obtained and by maintaining a suitable atmosphere. This includes a relaxed, nonhurried attitude on the part of the nurse, the relief of any discomfort or pain in the patient, a diminished noise level, a comfortable room temperature, and adequate lighting.

Assessment is a dynamic process. It begins with a thorough initial physical examination and interview, including a nursing history. (See Fig. 1–1.) If the patient is in distress, much of the history may be obtained from the family (significant other); or the nurse may wait until the patient is more comfortable. Ongoing exploration and clarification of the patient's physical and psychosocial status is necessary throughout the remainder of the hospitalization. Assessment, then, should be repeated on a routine basis once during every shift or more often, as the patient's condition dictates.

PSYCHOSOCIAL ASSESSMENT

In the Coronary Care Unit, the purpose of psychosocial assessment is to assist the patient in coping with the stress and suffering associated with cardiac disease. The nurse's assessment of the patient's coping abilities should focus on the following areas.

Patient Behavior

Cardiac disease has an overall effect on the patient's behavior. Initially, the patient may appear to be in anxiety, denial,

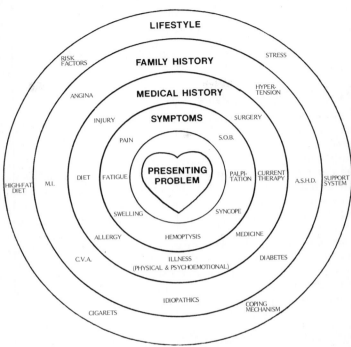

Figure 1–1. Components of nursing history for cardiac patients.

rationalization or aggressive sexual behavior. As the reality of the situation sets in, anger, depression, dependence or hypochondriasis may also appear.

Patient's Perception of Illness

The patient's perception of the illness may or may not correlate with the actual physical condition. Perception of the disease state is dependent upon the patient's

1. Understanding or knowledge of the illness (whether correct or not).
2. Immediate concerns. A problem at work or at home may be of higher priority.
3. Expected outcomes regarding the present illness and hospitalization. Included are the perceived impact of a coronary event on lifestyle, the symbolic meaning of heart disorders, fear of impending death and anxiety regarding the necessity for and length of a hospital stay.

4. Personal lifestyle. This includes the patient's occupation, marital situation, recreational habits, cultural beliefs, religious beliefs, habitual manner of dealing with stress, previous health behavior and preconceived ideas about health professionals.

Available Support Systems

The effect of cardiac illness on the patient is influenced by its effect on the family (significant other). All concerned may fear a resultant alteration in their interrelationships, levels of responsibility or financial status. It is of paramount importance to allow the frequent presence of loved ones as desired by the patient or as dictated by his physical condition. Religion may also play a major role in enabling the patient and family to adapt to the cardiac illness. The individual nurse's reaction to the patient as a unique human being rather than as someome with a diseased heart provides extra support. In addition, that the entire staff should be aware of the patient's potential for social isolation in an abundantly machined, stark, crisis-like atmosphere, full of strange noises and rigid procedures, cannot be overemphasized.

PHYSIOLOGICAL ASSESSMENT

Subjective Findings

These include symptoms described by the patient during the admission interview or daily assessment. The common symptoms of cardiac patients described as follows are usually caused by one or all of three physiological disorders: cardiac ischemia, pump insufficiency and rhythm disturbances.

Chest Pain.   This is caused by an O_2 supply inadequate to myocardial O_2 demand. It is a cardinal symptom of heart disease. The following elements of pain are usually assessed to confirm ischemic cardiac pain and to differentiate angina from myocardial infarction.

Characteristics.   Chest pain may be described as a "strange feeling," discomfort, dull heavy pressure, indigestion, crushing, burning, constricting, acting, stabbing and tightness.

Location.   Pain may be substernal, precordial, across the chest or around the nipple line. It may be diffused or localized.

Radiation.   The pain may also radiate to the jaw, teeth,

neck, left shoulder, left arm or both arms and the back. In some patients, the radiated pain rather than the chest pain is the only presenting discomfort.

Severity. Using a scale of 1 (least severe) to 10 (most severe), ask the patient to indicate the intensity of the pain. The recorded scale is used as a frame of reference to compare with future episodes.

Duration. This is defined as the exact time period of a continuous pain episode, which may last from minutes to hours. Several intermittent small episodes, however, are not considered a long pain period.

Precipitating and Aggravating Factors. Such factors include exertion, emotional excitement, nervousness, extreme coldness, deep breathing, position changes and deep sleep; or the pain may occur spontaneously without apparent precipitating factors.

Accompanying Symptoms. These may be anxiousness, shortness of breath, palpitation, sweating, nausea or vomiting.

Alleviating Factors. These include resting, sublingual nitroglycerine, O_2 administration and change of position. Pain lasting more than 20 minutes without relief is usually suggestive of myocardial infarction (MI).

Fatigue. This is caused by decreased cardiac output and inadequate O_2 supply to the myocardium. It is a common complaint of cardiac patients, especially when heart failure is present. The patient usually experiences progressively decreased activity tolerance.

Shortness of Breath (SOB). In cardiac patients, this is usually due to pulmonary congestion caused by left ventricular myocardial failure or valvular disorders. It may occur at rest or with exertion, during day or night time (nocturnal), gradually or suddenly. SOB is usually accompanied by apprehensiveness. The nurse should ask the patient to compare the present level of SOB with the usual respiration effort and should also explore with the patient what factors help or hinder breathing.

Palpitation. This is a sensation of rapid heartbeats, skipping, irregularity, or pounding and is accompanied by anxiousness. Often it is caused by tachyarrhythmia or premature ventricular beats. However, with some patients it may be only imaginary. The onset and termination may be abrupt. The rhythm may be irregular or skipping.

Syncope. This is defined as the momentary loss of consciousness resulting from the reduction of brain perfusion. In cardiac patients, it is caused by a sudden decrease in cardiac output due to arrhythmias (Stokes-Adams attacks, sick sinus syndrome, and so on), aortic stenosis or idiopathic hypertrophic subaortic stenosis. The onset is abrupt and lasts only a few seconds. Careful history-taking helps to differentiate cardiac syncope from those caused by epilepsy, emotional disturbances, hyperventilation, volume depletion, positional changes and so forth.

Objective Findings

These include data obtained by observation, palpation, auscultation and percussion.

General Appearance. At a glance, the nurse should observe the patient's facial expression, affect, level of consciousness, tone of voice, posture, movements, respiration rate and pattern, skin color and turgor, status in regard to diaphoresis and cachexia, nutritional state and reaction to the surroundings. All of these provide an initial composite picture of the patient and indicate the level of comfort or distress, as well as the nature, severity and duration of the cardiac illness.

Inspection of Neck Veins. The distensibility of the neck veins reflects the pressure and volume changes of the right atrium. Therefore, the purpose of neck vein inspection is to estimate central venous pressure (CVP) and to evaluate the pressure wave forms. The right internal rather than the external jugular vein has been found to be more reliable for both purposes.

Method of Inspection. Observation of the venous pulsation is best accomplished by shining a flashlight tangentially across the skin over the vein. In normal individuals, the maximum pulsation (meniscus of the blood column) is observed when the trunk of the body is inclined less than 30 degrees. In patients with elevated venous pressure, it may be necessary to elevate the head and trunk to as much as 90 degrees.

Method of Central Venous Pressure Estimation (Figure 1–2). The normal CVP is 4 to 10 cm of H_2O.

1. Elevate the patient's trunk to a position where the best venous pulsation can be observed.
2. Use the sternal angle (manubrial joint) as a reference point (about 4 to 5 cm above the center of the right atrium).

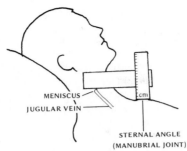

Figure 1–2. Method of central venous pressure estimation.

3. Measure the vertical distance between the sternal angle and the top of the oscillating venous column (meniscus). The value obtained in normal individuals should be less than 3 cm with the head of the bed at 30 to 45 degrees. Therefore, the CVP equals 3 cm + 4 to 5 cm = 7 to 8 cm H_2O. An elevation of CVP indicates increased right ventricular diastolic pressure due to right heart failure, tricuspid regurgitation, or tamponade. An extremely low CVP may indicate hypovolemia in patients with low output failure.

Meaning of Venous Pressure Wave Forms (Fig. 1–3). These wave forms represent phasic pressure changes in the right atrium. These consist of three positive waves and two troughs. It is suggested that the nurse listen to the heart sound while

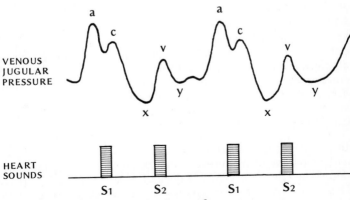

Figure 1–3. Wave forms of venous pressure.

assessing the change of wave forms and look for absent or unusually prominent waves.

a wave. This is the first positive wave and the most prominent, especially during inspiration. It is produced by atrial contraction and almost coincides with S_1. A large "a" wave indicates atrial contraction against increased resistance, such as in tricuspid stenosis, cor pulmonale, and so on. An irregular, enlarged "a" wave suggests atrioventricular (AV) dissociation. In atrial fibrillation, the "a" wave is absent.

c wave. A small positive wave may be visible at times. It is a reflected wave from the adjacent carotid artery.

x descent. This is the first trough, caused by atrial relaxation and the resulting fall of atrial pressure. It begins with ventricular systole and is between S_1 and S_2.

v wave. This is the third positive wave, caused by atrial filling from systemic venous return. It begins during the latter part of ventricular systole and almost coincides with S_2. A large "v" wave characterizes tricuspid valve regurgitation.

y descent. This is the second trough, produced by falling atrial pressure. During early diastole, the tricuspid valve opens and allows blood to flow rapidly into the ventricle.

Hepatojugular Reflex. This is present when venous pressure is elevated enough to cause liver engorgement. It is detected by positioning the patient so that the venous pulsation can be best observed (usually 45 degrees). Firm manual pressure is then applied over the right upper quadrant for 30 to 60 seconds. Observe the change in neck vein distention. When the meniscus increases more than 1 cm, it is considered to be a positive sign.

Palpation of the Carotid Arteries. This procedure is used for indirect assessment of cardiac activity, such as stroke volume and aortic competency. With fingertips, gently palpate the carotid artery one side at a time. The rate, rhythm, amplitude and contour of the pulse should be checked and compared. A bruit (a blowing sound) may be heard by listening to the carotid arteries with the diaphragm of a stethoscope. A bruit usually indicates a narrowing of the carotid artery or a radiation of an aortic valve murmur.

Inspection and Palpation of the Precordium. Inspection and palpation of the precordium are performed together to determine the presence of normal and abnormal pulsations. It is a useful method in assessing left, right and combined ventricular hypertrophy and is best performed using tangential lighting with the patient in a supine position. A left lateral position can be assumed by the patient to accentuate precordial movements. The examiner should stand at the patient's right side and observe the chest for size and symmetry and then for any pulsations, lifts, heaves or retractions. Palpation confirms observed phenomenon and is performed using the fingers and palmar aspect of the right hand.

Apical Impulse (Point of Maximal Impulse, PMI).   In about half of the normal adult population, a visible pulsation may be observed in the area of the midclavicular line in the fifth left intercostal space. Normally, it corresponds with ventricular systole and is a single, faint, instantaneous "tap" approximately 2 cm in diameter. In the presence of left ventricular hypertrophy or dilation and aneurysm, the apical impulse may be larger in size and more laterally or inferiorly located.

Retractions.   Marked or actual retraction of a rib just medial to the left midclavicular line in the fifth intercostal space is abnormal and may result from pericardial disease.

Heaves (Lifts).   A diffuse lifting impulse observed along the left sternal border or at the apex implies an increased contact of right ventricle or left ventricle with chest wall as found with dilatation-hypertrophy associated with various disorders (such as valvular diseases or pulmonary hypertension).

Thrills.   The abnormal turbulent blood flow causing an audible murmur of Grade V or VI intensity also results in palpable thrills. A thrill is best felt with the cupped palm and heel of the hand placed over the left precordium. It is similar to the rushing sensation felt when fingers are placed over the larynx of a purring cat. It may occur as a result of severe mitral regurgitation or a ruptured ventricular septum.

Auscultation of the Precordium

The Stethoscope.   This instrument gathers and slightly amplifies sound before it is transmitted to the ears. It should be equipped with both a bell and a diaphragm. The bell is applied lightly to the skin (so as not to stretch the skin) and is used to detect low-pitched (frequency) sounds such as gallops and diastolic murmurs. The diaphragm, however, should be placed firmly on the skin and detects high-pitched sounds such as systolic murmurs.

The Environment.   The surroundings should be warm and quiet. The patient's position should initially be supine. A left lateral recumbent position is used when there is suspicion of

ventricular gallops or mitral stenosis. Having the patient
assume an upright, sitting position and lean forward with
breath held on expiration is preferred when assessing for
early diastolic murmurs.

A Systematic Approach.   This is essential. A recommended
method is to begin auscultation at the base of the heart, at
the right second intercostal space, and then slowly move the
stethoscope down toward the apex. Pay special attention to
the precordial locations diagrammed in Figure 1–4. In aus-
cultating each area, concentrate on one component of the
cardiac cycle at a time—the first heart sound and then the
second heart sound. Listen carefully, noting the quality (crisp
or muffled), intensity (loud or soft), rhythm (irregular or
regular) and the presence of extra sounds (murmurs, gallops,
rubs or clicks). A pulse deficit is assessed by taking apical and
radial pulses simultaneously, noting differences in rate. Murmurs are common, and detection often requires a trained ear.
Specifics for murmur assessment are outlined in Table 1–1.
The origin of various abnormal heart sounds and their method
of assessment are described in Table 1–2.

Auscultation of Lung Sounds.   The auscultation of lung
sounds is an essential component of cardiovascular assessment
and provides information about cardiac function, especially
left ventricular performance. The patient should be instructed
to breathe deeply and slowly through an open mouth. With

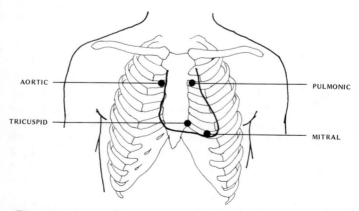

Figure 1–4.   Auscultation locations of heart sounds on the precordium.

Table 1–1. ASSESSMENT OF MURMURS

NOTE THE FOLLOWING CHARACTERISTICS:

1. Timing and duration of maximal intensity:
   Systolic: early, mid or late systole
                   midsystolic ejection vs. pansystolic (holosystolic)
   Diastolic: early, mid or late diastole
2. Quality: blowing, harsh, rumbling
3. Pitch: high, heard best with the diaphragm
   Low, heard best with the bell
4. Location: Where heard the loudest; 3rd or 4th left intercostal space, apical area or base of heart
5. Radiation: transmission of sound
6. Intensity (not necessarily equal to degree of disease):
   Grade I   Faint, not heard with every beat
   Grade II   Soft, but heard with every beat
   Grade III Moderately loud without accompanying thrill
   Grade IV Loud with possible palpable thrill
   Grade V   Very loud, heard only with the stethoscope and accompanied by a thrill
   Grade VI Very loud, heard without the stethoscope and accompanied by a thrill

the diaphragm of the stethoscope placed firmly on the skin, the lungs should be systematically auscultated, starting at the base (at about the tenth thoracic vertebrae) and then, moving in a zigzag pattern up the left and right posterior, lateral and anterior chest wall. One complete breathing cycle should be heard at each site of stethoscope placement, with analysis and comparison of breath sounds. Pitch, quality, intensity and duration of the inspiratory and expiratory phases should be noted. Table 1–3 briefly outlines normal and common abnormal findings.

Assessment of the Abdomen

Inspection. On inspection, the abdomen should be symmetrical in contour and should appear flat or slightly rounded. A distended abdomen may result from fluid (ascites), adipose tissue, gas, feces or malignancy and warrants further investigation. Dullness to percussion occurs over visceral organs, masses or fluid. Tympany (a hollow sound) is heard over a gas-filled bowel. The patient is best assessed in a supine position. Ascites is indicated when percussion yields dullness in the lateral flank areas with tympany heard medially.

Auscultation. This should precede percussion, as the latter stimulates bowel motility. Using the diaphragm of the steth-

Text continued on page 21

Table 1-2. HEART SOUNDS AND THEIR ASSESSMENT

TYPE OF HEART SOUND	ORIGIN	PREFERRED METHOD OF AUSCULTATION
I. S_1		
A. Normal S_1	S_1 is the first sound heard. It results from closure of the mitral and tricuspid valves (AV valves) and reflects ventricular contraction (systole). Tricuspid closure is often a quieter component of S_1.	Using the diaphragm of the stethoscope, S_1 is heard loudest at the apex and left lower sternal border.
B. Augmented S_1	S_1 is augmented when the mitral valve is still wide open at the onset of systole, causing it to slam shut. This occurs during sinus tachycardia and in mitral stenosis.	Same as above; however, S_1 is the same or louder than S_2 at the base.
C. Decreased S_1	S_1 is decreased when the mitral valve has "floated" back to a nearly closed position prior to ventricular contraction. This occurs in first-degree AV block and from mitral valve calcification, as in mitral regurgitation.	At the apex, S_1 has the same or less intensity as S_2.
D. Varying S_1	S_1 varies in intensity when the mitral valve is in varying position at the onset of ventricular contraction. This occurs in complete AV block and atrial fibrillation.	At any point on the precordium, the intensity of S_1 will vary from beat to beat.

E. Split S_1

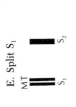

S_1 splitting may occur over the tricuspid area as the faint tricuspid component becomes more audible. This is a normal occurrence, as the left ventricle usually contracts slightly before the right ventricle, causing mitral valve closure to precede tricuspid valve closure.

S_1 splitting is best heard over the tricuspid area. If heard well over the apex, it is likely due to an S_4, or to an early systolic ejection click instead.

II. S_2

A. Normal S_2

S_2 results from the closure of the aortic and pulmonic valves and precedes diastole.

It is heard loudest using the diaphragm of the stethoscope at the base or pulmonic area of the heart.

B. S_2 with physiological splitting

Expiration

Inspiration

S_2 physiological splitting is a normal variation. Because right ventricular ejection time is longer than that of the left ventricle, pulmonic closure is slightly later than aortic closure. With inspiration, venous return is increased to the right ventricle, thus exaggerating the pulmonic delay.

Physiological splitting is best heard over the pulmonic area during the patient's inspiratory cycle.

C. S_2 with pathological splitting

1. Wide splitting

Expiration

Inspiration

Wide splitting of S_2 occurs when there is a marked delay in pulmonic valve closure due to pulmonic stenosis or right bundle branch block. It may also occur secondary to early closure of the aortic valve due to mitral regurgitation.

Wide splitting occurs throughout the respiratory cycle, increasing slightly on inspiration. It is best heard over the pulmonic area.

Table continued on following page

Table 1-2. HEART SOUNDS AND THEIR ASSESSMENT (Continued)

TYPE OF HEART SOUND	ORIGIN	PREFERRED METHOD OF AUSCULTATION
2. Fixed splitting *Expiration* *Inspiration* S_1 S_2 (AP) S_1 S_2 (AP)	Fixed splitting occurs as a result of an atrial septal defect and right ventricular failure.	Fixed splitting does not vary with respiration and is best heard over the pulmonic area.
3. Paradoxical splitting *Expiration* *Inspiration* S_1 S_2 (AP) S_1 S_2 (AP)	Paradoxical splitting occurs from delayed closure of the aortic valve. It may result from left bundle branch block or aortic stenosis.	Paradoxical splitting is best heard over the pulmonic area. A narrow split is heard during inspiration, with increased splitting noted during expiration.
D. Augmented S_2 S_1 S_2	S_2 is augmented due to the "slamming" shut of the aortic valve and occurs in arterial hypertension and aortic valve stenosis.	The intensity of S_2 is similar to or greater than S_1 at the apex.

E. Decreased S_2

S_1 S_2

S_2 is decreased in intensity when the aortic valve is calcified and, therefore, does not open widely during systole. This is seen in aortic stenosis.

S_2 is of decreased intensity when heard at the base of the heart.

III. Gallops: Diastolic Filling Sounds

A. S_3 (Ventricular gallop)
Systole—Diastole

S_1

S_2 S_3

S_3 occurs in early diastole during passive, rapid ventricular filling. Sudden changes of inflow volume cause vibrations of the valves and ventricular supporting structures. It is a normal variation in children and young adults. Heard in the older patient, it indicates increased myocardial failure and valvular incompetence.

S_3 is dull and low-pitched and occurs later than an opening snap. Using the bell, an S_3 due to left ventricular failure is best heard at the apex with the patient in a left lateral position. An S_3 due to right ventricular failure is best heard along the left lower sternal border in the supine position. The sound may be augmented during inspiration.

The bell is used to hear this low-pitched sound. It is best heard at or medial to the apex.

B. S_4 (Atrial gallop)
Systole—Diastole

S_4 S_1

S_2

S_4 occurs with atrial systole during active, rapid ventricular filling. When ventricular compliance is decreased, resistance to filling is increased, causing the ventricles and their supporting structures to vibrate during the "atrial kick." It is rarely heard in normal people. Its presence may result from myocardial infarction (transient), hypertension, cardiomyopathy, aortic stenosis, cor pulmonale or pulmonic stenosis. An S_4 is never heard in the absence of atrial contraction (i.e., atrial fibrillation).

Table continued on following page

Table 1-2. HEART SOUNDS AND THEIR ASSESSMENT (Continued)

TYPE OF HEART SOUND	ORIGIN	PREFERRED METHOD OF AUSCULTATION
C. Summation gallop S_1 S_3S_4 S_2	Summation gallops (quadruple rhythm) result when both phases of rapid ventricular filling become audible as S_3 and S_4. Increased heart rates can shorten diastole, making both sounds appear as one sound during diastole.	Summation gallops contain three cardiac sounds: S_1, S_2 and a summation sound of S_3 and S_4. It sounds very much like a horse's gallop and can be heard best at the apex.
IV. Other Extra Heart Sounds		
A. Opening snaps S_1 S_2 OS	Opening snaps occur early in diastole and are brief, high-pitched sounds of a snapping or clicking quality. They are associated with the opening of a stenotic mitral valve and (rarely) tricuspid valve. They are usually accompanied by a loud S_1 and are more easily detected when higher left atrial pressures exist.	Opening snaps are best heard with the diaphragm of the stethoscope at the apex. The sound radiates rather widely.
B. Ejection click 1. Early systolic S_1 EC S_2	Ejection clicks occur early, mid or late in systole. Early systolic ejection clicks occur early in systole with the opening of the semilunar valves and are associated with a dilated aorta or pulmonary artery, a stenotic aortic valve or pulmonic valve and pulmonary hypertension. Mid to late ejection clicks are often related to a ballooning deformity of the mitral valve and are accompanied by late systolic murmurs.	Aortic ejection clicks are most common and are heard with the diaphragm of the stethoscope at both the base and the apex. There is no variation with respiration. Pulmonic ejection clicks are best assessed over the pulmonic valve. A decreased intensity of the click during inspiration is characteristic.

2. Mid to late systolic click

V. Murmurs
A. Systolic murmurs
1. Ejection type

Systolic ejection murmurs are associated with forward blood flow during ventricular contraction across stenotic aortic or pulmonic valves.

Use of the stethoscope diaphragm is indicated. Ejection murmurs are typically of medium pitch and harsh quality and may be associated with an early ejection click. Aortic ejection murmurs are best heard over the aortic valve with radiation into the neck, down the left sternal border and occasionally to the apex. They may be accompanied by a decreased S_2. Pulmonic ejection murmurs are heard best over the pulmonic valve, with radiation toward the left shoulder and left neck vessels. These murmurs may be accompanied by a wide split S_2.

Table continued on following page

Table 1–2. HEART SOUNDS AND THEIR ASSESSMENT (Continued)

TYPE OF HEART SOUND	ORIGIN	PREFERRED METHOD OF AUSCULTATION
2. Pansystolic regurgitant murmurs	Pansystolic murmurs occur when blood regurgitates through incompetent mitral and tricuspid valves (AV valves) or a ventricular septal defect as pressures rise during systole and blood seeks chambers of lower pressure. Damage to valve leaflets, papillary muscles and chordae tendinae result in mitral valve insufficiency (blood regurgitates from left ventricle to left atrium) and tricuspid valve insufficiency (blood regurgitates from the right ventricle to right atrium). A ventricular septal defect results in blood regurgitation from the left ventricle to the right ventricle.	All regurgitant murmurs are high pitched, and those of AV valve incompetence have a blowing quality. Mitral regurgitant murmurs are heard at the apex with radiation into the left axilla and may be accompanied by an ejection click and signs of left ventricular failure. Tricuspid regurgitant murmurs are heard loudest over the tricuspid area, with radiation into the sternum. Ventricular septal defects are usually loud, harsh and heard best over the left sternal border in the fourth, fifth and sixth intercostal spaces with radiation over the precordium but not the axilla.
3. Early systolic murmurs	Early systolic murmurs (innocent murmurs) are associated with high cardiac outputs, as there is increased blood flow velocity across normal semilunar valves. Causes include anemia, tachycardia, thyrotoxicosis and fever. The murmur will disappear with correction of the underlying condition. These are a normal variant in children.	These murmurs are best heard with the bell over the base of the heart or along the lower left sternal border. They are usually no greater than a Grade II, are of medium pitch and have a blowing quality. Intensity may increase during inspiration with the patient in a left recumbent position or with increased heart rates.

4. Late systolic murmurs

Late systolic murmurs imply mild mitral regurgitation as the mitral valve balloons into the left atrium late in ventricular systole.

It is best heard with the diaphragm of the stethoscope over the apex and is often preceded by a mid or late systolic ejection click.

B. Diastolic murmurs
1. Early diastolic murmur

Early diastolic murmurs (decrescendo murmurs) are usually caused by semilunar valve insufficiency, with regurgitation due to valvular deformity or dilation of the valvular ring. They are heard immediately following the second heart sound and then diminish in intensity as the pressure in the aorta or pulmonary artery falls and the ventricles fill.

These murmurs are heard best with the diaphragm at the base of the heart with the patient leaning forward in deep expiration. They are high-pitched and blowing and radiate down the left sternal border, perhaps to the apex or down the right sternal border. Accompanying signs of heart failure may be present.

2. Diastolic filling rumbling

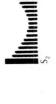

Diastolic filling rumbles are caused as blood flows across stenotic AV valves (more often mitral). They may also occur during augmented blood flow across normal AV valves. The murmur has two phases, becoming louder as the blood flow from the atrium to the ventricle increases and passive ventricular filling just after AV valve opening and again during atrial contraction (presystole).

With the bell, this murmur is heard over only a small area at and just medial to the apex. Exercise and a left lateral position of the patient increase the intensity of the sound. It is a low-pitched, rumbling sound often accompanied by an augmented S_1 and an opening snap.

Table continued on following page

Table 1–2. HEART SOUNDS AND THEIR ASSESSMENT (Continued)

TYPE OF HEART SOUND	ORIGIN	PREFERRED METHOD OF AUSCULTATION
VI. Combined Systolic-Diastolic Heart Sounds		
A. Friction rub 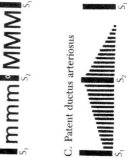	Friction rubs are produced by inflammation of the pericardial sac (pericarditis) as the roughened parietal and visceral layers of the pericardium rub against each other. There are three components of this sound that correspond with cardiac activity: (1) ventricular systole, (2) ventricular diastole and (3) atrial systole. One or all three components may be heard.	Friction rubs are a to-and-fro, scratchy, grating, "squeaky leather" sound that may seem close to the ear. All three components clearly differentiate this sound from the two-component pleural friction rub. The diaphragm of the stethoscope picks up this high-pitched sound at the apex and upper left sternal border (third intercostal space) and is loudest with the patient leaning forward in exhalation.
B. Venous hum	Venous hums are nonpathological sounds produced by turbulent blood flow in the internal jugular veins of many children and some adults. It is a continuous sound heard loudest during diastole.	A venous hum is a low-pitched, slightly roaring sound heard above the medial clavicular area, especially on the right side. It is best assessed with the patient sitting upright and increases in intensity as the head is turned to the left and slightly upward. Mild pressure on the jugular veins will obliterate the sound.
C. Patent ductus arteriosus	Patent ductus arteriosus (PDA) murmurs result from the presence of a congenitally abnormal communication channel between the aorta and the pulmonary artery. It is a continuous murmur heard loudest during late systole, fading by mid to late diastole.	This loud murmur, often accompanied by a thrill, is easily detected over the pulmonic area with radiation toward the left clavicle. It is a very harsh sound of medium pitch.

oscope, bowel tones should be assessed in all four abdominal quadrants. High-pitched gurgling sounds are normally heard every 5 to 15 seconds. At least 5 minutes of auscultation are recommended to determine the presence of bowel sounds. Decreased motility accompanies electrolyte disturbances, paralytic ileus, peritonitis, bowel manipulation and pneumonia. Increased motility results from laxative use and gastroenteritis. Loud bruits heard with the bell just over or above the umbilicus may herald the presence of an aortic obstruction. Murmurs heard over the upper midline or toward the flank arise from renal arterial stenosis.

Assessment of Periphery

Skin. As the body's largest organ, the skin reflects changes in the internal environment and provides valuable information regarding cardiovascular performance.

Color. Cyanosis, a dusky blue color, may be observed in the lips, oral mucosa, nail beds and ear lobes. It results from increased amounts of reduced hemoglobin (deoxygenation) of venous blood seen in severe pulmonary disease and cardiovascular incompetence. Pallor is observed as peripheral blood flow diminishes or hemoglobin decreases. Mottling of the skin results from a combination of arteriolar constriction and venous stasis.

Temperature. Skin temperature reflects blood flow to the dermis. Decreased cardiac output and shock result in generalized hypothermia. Moist, clammy skin results from an outpouring of catecholamines in response to stress.

Hair Distribution. Chronic arterial insufficiency causes the skin of the legs and feet to become hairless and to appear atrophic and shiny.

Clubbing. A chronic decrease in oxygenation may result in clubbing of the fingers ("drumstick fingers"). Nails become wide and flattened and lie at an angle of 180 degrees or more to the nail base. Causes include cardiovascular and pulmonary diseases and liver cirrhosis.

Turgor. Skin elasticity is determined by picking up a fold of skin and observing how quickly it returns to its normal shape. Loss of turgor reflects an extracellular volume deficit or the normal changes that occur with aging and chronic steroid use.

Stasis Dermatitis. Chronic venous and arterial insufficiency may result in ulcer formation in the lower leg, ankle

Table 1–3.   LUNG SOUNDS

TYPES	DESCRIPTIONS
I. Normal breath sounds	
A. Vesicular 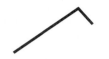 *Inspiration Expiration*	Vesicular sounds are normal breath sounds heard over lung parenchyma. They are low in pitch and intensity, composed of a louder, longer inspiratory phase (5:2) than expiratory phase.
B. Bronchovesicular	Bronchovesicular sounds are normal findings in the areas of major bronchi. They are characterized by equal inspiratory and expiratory phases. These moderately pitched sounds are heard at the first and second intercostal space and along the sternal border. If heard over peripheral lung fields, it may indicate consolidation of lung tissue.
C. Bronchial (tubular)	Bronchial sounds are high pitched and normally heard over the trachea. They have a longer expiratory phase with a short gap between phases. If heard over lung tissue, this sound may indicate consolidation of lung tissue.
II. Abnormal (adventitious) breath sounds	
A. Rales	Rales are noncontinuous crackling sounds that can be simulated by rubbing hair together near the ear. They are produced as air passes through secretions in the tracheobronchial tree and alveoli or as alveoli, closed during expiration, suddenly open during inspiration. Distribution, intensity and duration of rales vary according to the site of production and quality of secretions. Fine rales usually indicate increased moisture in small passages and alveoli. Medium-to-coarse rales result from moisture in the bronchi within the bronchi and bronchioles. Conditions causing rales include congestive heart failure, pulmonary fibrosis, atelectasis and pneumonia. If they are heard, the patient should be asked to cough, and the lung area should be reassessed for clearing.

Table 1–3. LUNG SOUNDS (*Continued*)

TYPES	DESCRIPTIONS
B. Rhonchi	Rhonchi are continuous sounds produced as air passes through a tracheobronchial tree (partially obstructed or narrowed). They can occur in either inspiratory or expiratory phases or in both but are more common in the expiratory, as bronchi are shortened and narrowed during this phase. *High-pitched rhonchi* have a wheezing quality that often increases with forced expiration. They generally originate in smaller bronchi and bronchioles. *Low-pitched rhonchi* have a snoring (sonorous) quality and result from partial obstruction of the larger bronchi or trachea.
C. Pleural friction rub 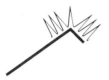	Pleural friction rubs are dry, creaking, grating sounds produced by the rubbing together of inflamed and roughened pleural layers during the respiratory cycle. The sound is heard in both the inspiratory and the expiratory phase. It is heard best at the lower anterolateral thorax, as thoracic expansion is greatest there. Coughing does not alter the sound.
D. Diminished breath sounds 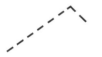	Diminished or absent breath sounds may occur over areas in the tracheobronchial tree and among alveoli that are collapsed or occluded (atelectasis, pneumothorax). Decreased air velocity through air passages, as in emphysema, may produce decreased breath sounds. Any decrease in chest wall movement over the abnormal site should be noted.

and foot. Edema, brown pigmentation and cyanosis of the foot on dependency often accompanies ulcers of venous insufficiency. Pallor of the foot with elevation and rubor during dependency accompanies ulcers of arterial insufficiency.

Edema.   Abnormal fluid collection within the interstitium or body cavities may be caused by an increase in hydrostatic pressure (heart failure), decreases in plasma protein levels (liver and kidney disease) and insufficient venous or lymphatic return. Dependent edema is commonly assessed for in the ankles, pretibial area and sacrum. To test for pitting, press edematous area with a finger. If an indentation remains, pitting edema is present.

Blood Pressure.   Blood pressure is that pressure exerted by plasma and blood cells against the arterial walls, with its peak in systole and trough in diastole. The sounds arise from turbulent blood flow through an artery constricted by external pressure (inflated cuff). The size of the cuff used should be about 20 per cent wider than the diameter of the desired limb and long enough to encircle it. A cuff too small results in falsely high pressure, whereas large cuffs cause false low readings. If arms are inaccessible, pressure can be obtained using the thighs and popliteal artery or the calves and posterior tibial artery. Systolic pressures may be obtained through palpation if pressures are hard to auscultate. Blood pressure should be initially measured in both arms to rule out dissecting aortic aneurysm, vascular obstruction and so forth.

Pulse Pressure.   The difference between systolic and diastolic pressures is the pulse pressure, and it reflects stroke volume. A normal pulse pressure is 30 to 40 mm Hg. A widened pulse pressure occurs in high cardiac output states such as thyrotoxicosis, fever, anemia and aortic regurgitation. Causes of a decreased pulse pressure include shock, aortic stenosis and cardiac tamponade, or nitroglycerine effect.

Pulsus Paradoxicus.   The cuff should be slowly deflated as the patient breathes slowly and deeply. The first sound of systole is noted, and the cuff is slowly deflated until sounds can be heard throughout the respiratory cycle. This point should be noted. An auscultatory gap in systolic pressure of 10 mm Hg or greater during inspiration is considered abnormal. Causes include pericardial tamponade, pulmonary hypertension, and asthma.

Orthostatic Hypotension.   If there is any suspicion of extracellular volume depletion or decreased vascular tone, the blood pressure should be taken in a supine position and then in a sitting or standing position. An abnormal orthostatic drop is considered to be 10 to 15 mm Hg for systolic pressure and 10 mm Hg for diastolic. It is often accompanied by a compensatory increase in the pulse rate of 10 to 20 per cent.

Pulses.   Palpation of pulses is performed by placing the first three fingers along the length of the desired artery. Press gently against the bone or firm surface and gradually release pressure. The radial, carotid, femoral, posterior tibial, dorsalis pedis and abdominal aortic pulses should be palpated routinely. The brachial and popliteal arteries may be assessed if more distal pulses are not present. Rate, rhythm and amplitude should be noted, along with bilateral pressures.

Waterhammer Pulse.   This is a large, bounding pulse with rapid rises and falls and is associated with wide pulse pressures.

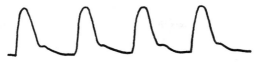

Pulsus Tardus.   This is a weak pulse with a slow upstroke and prolonged peak and is associated with decreased pulse pressure.

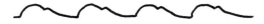

Pulsus Alternans.   This is a pulse that has a normal rhythm but alternates in amplitude from beat to beat and is seen in myocardial failure.

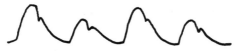

Bigeminal Pulse.   This is a rhythm disturbance produced by a normal (strong) beat alternating with a premature contraction (weak). The irregularity of the pulse differentiates if from pulsus alternans.

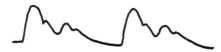

Miscellaneous
Urinary Output.   This decreases when cardiac output falls low enough to reduce the renal perfusion. It should be maintained at a minimum of 20 to 30 ml per hour. Continuous reduction of urinary output in cardiac patients is one of the early signs of heart failure or impending shock.

Body Weight.   This should be measured on admission and daily as soon as the patient's intake and output record is no longer maintained. It is a sensitive method for detecting sodium and water retention even before edema is evident. For the purpose of having an accurate comparison, the body weight should be obtained at the same time each day (ideally before breakfast) with the same amount of clothing or bedding. A shift of the body weight of 3 lb or more within 24 hours is generally considered to result from water rather than body mass changes.

SUGGESTED READINGS

Bates, B.: *A Guide to Physical Examination,* 2nd ed. Philadelphia, J. B. Lippincott, 1979.

Benjamin, A.: *The Helping Interview.* Boston, Houghton Mifflin, 1969.

Bogdonoff, M. D.: Psychological impact of coronary care unit. In *Advanced Cardiac Nursing.* Bowie, Maryland, The Charles Press Publishers, 1970.

Borg, N. (ed.): *Core Communication for Critical Care Nursing,* 2nd ed. American Association of Critical Care Nurses. Philadelphia, W. B. Saunders, 1981.

Brammer, L. M.: *The Helping Relationship Process and Skills.* Englewood Cliffs, N.J., Prentice-Hall, 1973.

Little, D., and Carnevali, D. L.: *Nursing Care Planning.* Philadelphia, J. B. Lippincott, 1976.

Malasanos, L., et al.: *Health Assessment,* 2nd ed. St. Louis, C. V. Mosby, 1981.

Scalzi, C. C.: Nursing management of behavioral responses following an acute myocardial infarction. *Heart and Lung,* 2:62, 1973.

II

DIAGNOSTIC TESTS

2

ELECTROCARDIOGRAPHY AND CARDIAC MONITORING

DEFINITIONS

Polarized State

The cell is at rest in a polarized state. Although the inside of the cell is negative with respect to the outside, its membrane remains electrically intact. The membrane resting potential (MRP) is −90 mv.

Depolarization

Depolarization is the propagation of an electrical impulse due to an abrupt change in the permeability of the cell membrane, allowing the inside of the cell to become increasingly positive with respect to the outside (Na enters the cell and K leaves).

Repolarization

The cell returns to its resting state (Na leaves the cell and K enters).

Electrocardiogram (EKG, ECG)

An electrocardiogram is a recorded graph of waves that represent variations in the time sequence of the electrical potentials produced by depolarization and repolarization of the myocardium.

Electrocardiography

Electrocardiography is the science of taking and interpreting electrocardiograms in order to diagnose cardiac disease by consistent correlation of characteristic patterns.

RATIONALE

The movement of ions that produces the depolarization and repolarization of the myocardium can be detected on the body surface. Electrodes placed upon the surface of the body will pick up various components of this ionic movement. By connecting these electrodes to an ECG machine, the electrical potentials of the heart are recorded and depicted as wave forms. An upright deflection represents a positive electrical potential and occurs when the current travels toward the recording electrode. A downward deflection represents a negative electrical potential and occurs when the current travels away from the recording electrode.

INDICATIONS

Arrhythmia
Chest pain
Myocardial infarction
Determination of heart rate
Chamber dilation or hyper-
    trophy

Pericarditis
Effect of drugs (especially
    cardiac)
Electrolyte disturbances (es-
    pecially K)
Effect of certain systemic
    diseases on the heart

LIMITATIONS

The ECG should always be correlated with the patient's clinical assessment. A patient with a normal heart may show nonspecific ECG changes, whereas a patient with a diseased heart may have a normal ECG.

ECG GRID

An ECG grid (Fig. 2–1) is a graph that allows for measurement of electrical activity during the cardiac cycle. The horizontal axis represents time, whereas the vertical axis represents voltage. All fine horizontal and vertical lines are present at 1-mm intervals, with a heavier line present every 5 mm. The routine recording speed is 25 mm per second. Recording at 50 mm per second spreads the tracing out, whereas recording at 12.5 mm per second, pushes the complexes closer together than normal.

COMPONENTS OF THE ELECTROCARDIOGRAM

See Figure 2–2.

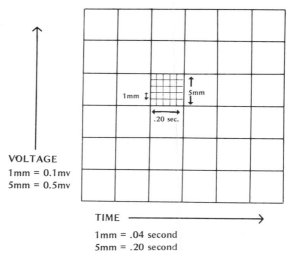

Figure 2–1. ECG grid.

P Wave

1. Represents atrial depolarization.
2. Contour.
   a. In leads I, II and AVF, it is upright, usually rounded, although it may be slightly pointed or slightly notched.
   b. In V_1 it may be diphasic or negative.
3. Normal range, lead II.
   a. Height is 0.3 mm to 2.0 mm.
   b. Duration is 0.05 second to 0.12 second.

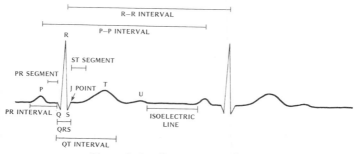

Figure 2–2. Components of ECG.

P-R Interval

1. Represents atrioventricular conduction time, including the normal delay in the atrioventricular (AV) junction of ± 0.07 second.
2. Measured from the beginning of the P wave to the beginning of the QRS complex.
3. Normal range is 0.12 second to 0.20 second.
4. The portion of this interval from the end of the P wave to the beginning of the QRS complex (P-R segment) is normally isoelectric.

QRS Complex

1. Represents ventricular depolarization.
2. Measured from the beginning of the Q wave (or R wave if no Q is present) to the end of the S wave.
3. Normal range is up to .11 second in duration.
4. Uppercase (capital) letters represent waves greater than 5 mm in height, while lowercase (small) letters represent waves less than 5 mm in height.

Definitions of Components of QRS.   See Figure 2–3.

   a. Q (q) is the initial negative deflection preceding the first positive deflection.
   b. R (r) is the first positive deflection, whether preceded by a Q or not.
   c. S (s) is the first negative deflection following the first positive deflection.
   d. R' (r') is the second positive deflection; it follows the S wave.
   e. S' (s') is the negative deflection following R'.

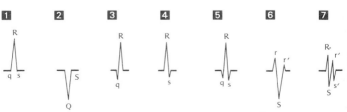

Figure 2–3.   Labeling the QRS complex.

QT Interval

1. Represents the duration of ventricular systole.
2. Measured from the beginning of the Q wave to the end of the T wave.
3. Normal range should be a corrected figure (QT_c), as it varies with heart rate.
   a. In women up to 0.43 second.
   b. In men up to 0.42 second.

J Point

This is the point marking the end of the QRS complex and the beginning of the ST segment.

ST Segment

1. Represents the time during which the ventricles remain in a depolarized state until the time ventricular repolarization begins.
2. Measured from the end of the S wave (J point) to the beginning of the T wave.
3. Normal range.
   a. Usually isoelectric.
   b. In precordial leads may vary from (-0.5 mm) to $+2.0$ mm from the baseline.
   c. In standard leads may vary from (-0.5 mm) to $+1.0$ mm from the baseline.

T Wave

1. Represents ventricular depolarization.
2. Contour.
   a. Normally upright in leads I, II and V_{3-6}.
   b. Slightly rounded and slightly asymmetrical.
3. Normal range.
   a. Standard limb leads, 1.0 to 5.0 mm in height.
   b. Precordial leads, no greater than 10 mm in height.
4. The supranormal refractory period of the cardiac action potential coincides with the downward slope of the T wave, during which time a weak stimulus can evoke an electrical response.

U Wave

1. Significance is not known; however, it may be noted in association with low serum potassium levels, high serum

calcium levels, bradycardia, left ventricular hypertrophy and subarachnoid hemorrhage.
2. Immediately follows the T wave and precedes the next P wave.
3. Same polarity as the T wave.
4. Normal range in height is not more than 1 mm.

T-P Interval

1. Represents the electrical resting potential of the heart.
2. Measured from the end of the T wave to the beginning of the P wave.
3. Contour is isoelectric and represents the baseline; i.e., elevations or depressions of other ECG componets are determined by comparison to the isoelectric line.
4. Normal range varies with the heart rate; i.e., the T-P interval shortens with tachycardias and lengthens with bradycardias.

P-P Interval

1. Represents atrial rate.
2. Measured as the distance between two successive P waves.

R-R Interval

1. Represents ventricular rate.
2. Measured as the distance between two successive R waves.
3. If rhythm is regular, R-R interval may be used to compute heart rate.

Abnormalities of ECG Components

See Table 2–1.

LEADS OF THE ELECTROCARDIOGRAM

Definition

A lead is defined as the connection of a positive and a negative electrode through an ECG machine (galvanometer) for continuous recording of the potential differences (voltages) between the two electrodes during the cardiac cycle.

Table 2–1. ABNORMALITIES OF ECG COMPONENTS

ECG COMPONENTS	SHORTENED	PROLONGED	ELEVATED OR WITH ↑ AMPLITUDE	INVERTED OR OF ↓ AMPLITUDE
P wave	—	Diseased or enlarged atrial muscle	Enlarged atria Notched, left at hypertrophy (P mitrale) Peaked, right at hypertrophy (P pulmonale)	Dextrocardia Low atrial rhythm Left atrial rhythm AV junctional rhythm
P-R interval	Low atrial rhythms AV junction rhythms Accelerated conduction	AV block, organic or drug induced (digitalis, Quinidine)	—	—
QRS complex	—	Hemiblock Bundle branch block Ventricular dysarrhythmia	Ventricular hypertrophy	Widespread myocardial damage Heart failure Pericardial effusion Myxedema

Q-T interval	Quinidine, procainamide Hypocalcemia Heart failure Myocardial infarction Cerebral disease (especially, subarachnoid hemorrhage) Rheumatic fever	Digitalis effect Hypercalcemia Hyperkalemia	—
ST segment	May be normal in healthy young blacks Pericarditis Myocarditis Myocardial injury Ventricular aneurysm Hyperkalemia Cerebrovascular accident (CVA)	Digitalis effect Bundle branch block Ventricular hypertrophy Myocardial ischemia	—
T wave	—	—	Ventricular hypertrophy Cerebral disease (especially, SAH) Myocardial ischemia

Types

Standard 12 Leads.   These include the standard and augmented limb leads and the precordial chest leads.

Standard Limb Leads.   Leads I, II and III are the standard limb leads. These are bipolar leads used to compare the electrical potential of a positive and a negative electrode, representing two limbs (except right leg). See Table 2–2.

Augmented Limb Leads.   Leads AVR, AVL and AVF are unipolar leads used to compare the electrical potential of an exploring electrode (positive) placed on one limb and a central terminal (negative), which represents an average potential (close to zero) of two other limbs. See Table 2–2.

Precordial (Chest) Leads.   Leads V_1, V_2, V_3, V_4, V_5, and V_6 (Fig. 2–4) are also unipolar leads used to compare the electrical potential of a positive exploring electrode (in various locations on the chest) and a central terminal (negative),

Table 2–2.   ELECTRODE PLACEMENT OF THE STANDARD 12 LEADS

TYPE OF LEADS	LOCATION OF (+) ELECTRODE	LOCATION OF (−) ELECTRODE	
Bipolar			
I	Left arm (LA)	Right arm (RA)	
II	Left Leg (LL)	Right arm (RA)	
III	Left Leg (LL)	Left arm (LA)	
Unipolar			
Augmented			
AVR	Right arm (RA)	Central* terminal	LA + LL
AVL	Left arm (LA)	is the average	RA + LL
AVF	Left leg (LL)	potential of two limbs	RA + LA
Precordial			
V_1	Fourth ICS† to the right of the sternum	Central terminal is the average potential of three limbs (RA, LA and LL). All six precordial leads use the same terminal.	
V_2	Fourth ICS to the left of the sternum		
V_3	Halfway between V_2 and V_4		
V_4	Fifth ICS in the midclavicular line		
V_5	Same level as V_4 in the anterior axillary line		
V_6	Same level as V_5 in the midaxillary line		

*Central terminal: The combination of electrodes is determined by the lead selector. (Modified from Phillips, R. E., and Feeney, M. K.: *The Cardiac Rhythms*, 2nd ed. Philadelphia, W. B. Saunders, 1980.)

† ICS, Intercostal space.

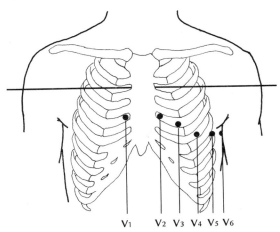

Figure 2–4. Precordial electrode placement.

which represents an average potential of right arm, left arm and left leg (See Table 2–2).

Miscellaneous Leads

Lewis Lead (L).   This is a special bipolar chest lead. The negative and positive electrodes are placed at the second and fourth intercostal spaces to the right of the sternum. The tracing is recorded on Lead I. It is used to amplify atrial waves and clarify the mechanism of atrial arrhythmias.

Esophageal Lead (E).   This is a unipolar lead. The exploring electrode is inserted via a nasal catheter located at various levels of the esophagus (20 cm, 40 cm, and so on). The central terminal is the same as in the precordial leads. It is used to explore atrial activity.

Intracardiac Lead.   This lead is the same as other unipolar leads except that the positive exploring electrode is inserted via cardiac catheterization and located in various chambers of the heart. It is used to record AV conduction and clarify the origin of arrhythmias.

Uses of the Standard 12 Leads.   The leads are used to explore electrical activity of the heart from various views as well as in the frontal and horizontal planes.

Views and Planes	*Leads*
Anteroseptal view	V_1, V_2, V_3, V_4
Anterolateral view	I, AVL, V_5, V_6
Diaphragmatic view	II, III, AVF
Intracavity view	AVR
Frontal plane	All standard and augmented limb leads
Horizontal plane	All precordial leads

VECTOR AND CARDIAC AXIS

Vector

In physics, it is an arrow that represents the magnitude and direction of a force. The length of the arrow indicates magnitude, and the arrowhead indicates direction. In the heart, a vector represents the electrical potential (force) produced by the myocardium and the direction toward which the electrical current is propagating. As illustrated in Figure 2–5, electrical forces propagate to various directions in the heart at a given moment. Forces of equal magnitude propagating in the opposite directions cancel each other out. Forces propagating in the same direction summate.

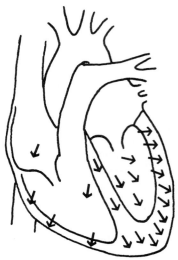

Figure 2–5. Electrical vectors in the heart.

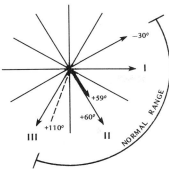

Figure 2–6.   Cardiac axis and its normal range.

Cardiac Axis (Mean Cardiac Vector)

The *net* or *resultant* electrical potential produced by the myocardium at a given moment is the cardiac axis. It is represented by the mean vector of QRS (ventricular depolarization), as the left ventricle constitutes the majority of muscle mass. The usual cardiac axis is located at or around +60 degrees in the frontal plane. However, it may range from −30 degrees to +110 degrees (Fig. 2–6).

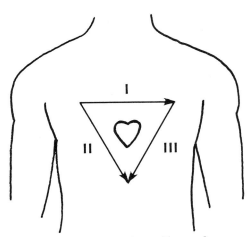

Figure 2–7.   Einthoven's triangle.

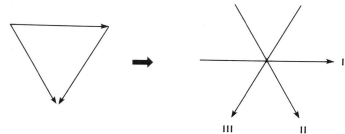

Figure 2–8. Triaxial figure.

DERIVATION OF HEXAXIAL FIGURE

Einthoven's Triangle

Einthoven's triangle is an equilateral triangle with the heart as a center point, formulated by a diagrammatical connection of electrodes from the standard limb leads. It is based on the assumption that Leads I, II and III are equally distant to the heart (Fig. 2–7).

Triaxial Figure

This figure is derived from Einthoven's triangle by shifting all sides (axes) of the equilateral triangle until they intersect at the same center point (Fig. 2–8). The head of the arrow represents the positive (+) pole of the lead, and the tail of the arrow is the negative pole (−). Lead I points to 0 degrees, Lead II to +60 degrees and Lead III to +120 degrees.

Hexaxial Figure

This figure is formulated by adding the three augmented limb leads to the triaxial figure (Fig. 2–9). The hexaxial figure is used to determine and depict the cardiac axis in the frontal

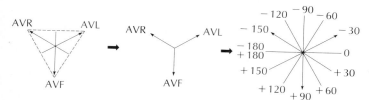

Figure 2–9. Hexaxial figure.

plane. The electrical field above Lead I is designated negative, and that below Lead I is positive. Therefore, AVL points to −30 degrees, AVR to +150 degrees and AVF to +90 degrees.

DETERMINATION OF CARDIAC AXIS IN THE FRONTAL PLANE

Purpose

Estimation of the Electrical Position of the Heart. If the axis is 0 to −30 degrees, the heart is horizontal. If the axis is +75 to +110 degrees, the heart is considered vertical.

Estimation of Axis Deviation. When the cardiac axis is between +110 and +180 degrees, it is called right axis deviation (RAD). RAD is often observed in patients with right bundle branch block (RBBB), right ventricular hypertrophy (RVH) and left posterior hemiblock (LPH). When the cardiac axis is between −30 and −90 degrees, it is called left axis deviation (LAD). LAD is often observed in patients with left bundle branch block (LBBB), left ventricular hypertrophy (LVH) and left anterior hemiblock (LAH).

Methods

Mathematical Method

a. Obtain the net amplitude of the QRS complex in two of the limb leads, such as Leads I and II in Figure 2–10.

b. Plot both amplitudes (+5 and +16) on the respective lead axis of a hexaxial figure at points A and B (Fig. 2–11).

c. Draw a perpendicular line on Lead I through point A and on Lead II through point B (Fig. 2–11).

d. The two perpendicular lines are intersected at point C. The resultant cardiac axis is the arrow between the center of the hexaxial figure and point C. Its angle is 75 degrees (Fig. 2–11).

Lead Reference Method. This method is used frequently in the clinical area for quick approximation of the cardiac axis. It is based on the principle that the cardiac axis is always parallel or nearly parallel to the lead with the largest net QRS

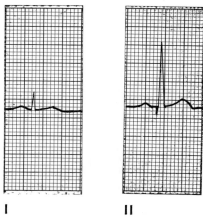

Figure 2–10. Net QRS amplitude: Lead I $= +5$, Lead II $= +16$
$(R - q = 18 - 2)$.

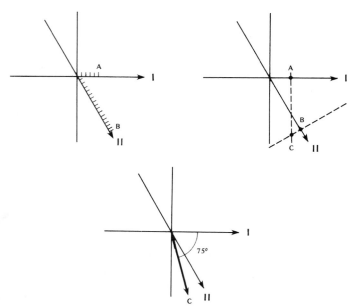

Figure 2–11. Estimation of cardiac axis.

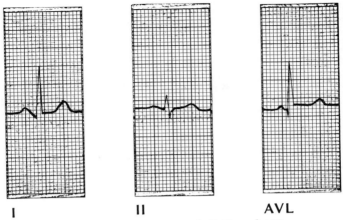

Figure 2–12. QRS in Leads I, II, and AVL.

amplitude and perpendicular or nearly perpendicular to the lead with zero or the smallest net QRS amplitude.

In Figure 2–12,

1. Lead II has the smallest net QRS amplitude (+1). Therefore, the cardiac axis must be nearly perpendicular to Lead II. The lead perpendicular to II is AVL.
2. Note that both Lead I and AVL have the largest net QRS amplitude. The cardiac axis must be nearly parallel to both I and AVL and equally close to both axes.
3. The cardiac axis, therefore, is around −15 degrees, which is between Lead I and AVL.

CALCULATION OF HEART RATE

If the rhythm is irregular, heart rate should be determined by counting the number of heartbeats (QRS) in a full-minute ECG strip. If the rhythm is regular, any of the following methods can be used.

1. Count the number of small squares in the ECG paper within one R-R interval and divide this number into 1500 (1-minute length of ECG paper consists of 1500 small squares).
2. Count the number of big squares within one R-R interval and divide this number into 300 (1-minute length of ECG

paper consists of 300 big squares). This method can be simplified by using the following formulas.

If the number of big squares between R-R is	*Heart rate should be*
1	300
2	150
3	100
4	75
5	60
6	50
7	43
8	37
9	33
10	30

3. Count the number of QRS complexes within a 6-second time period on the ECG strip and multiply by 10.

ANALYSIS OF ECG RHYTHM

A systematic approach to analysis is recommended to ensure accuracy and inclusiveness. The following items are suggested content. Analysis may begin with any of these steps. However, it should begin with the most striking feature noted.

1. Regularity of the rhythm (R-R interval).
2. Ventricular rate.
3. Width of the QRS complex.
4. Presence of P wave.
5. P-QRS relationship.
6. Regularity of P-P interval.
7. Atrial rate.
8. P-R interval and its consistency.
9. Consistency of the shapes and contours of the waves and complexes.

NORMAL SINUS RHYTHM (NSR)

ECG Criteria

Rate and Rhythm.   Rate is 60 to 100 beats per minute, and rhythm is regular.

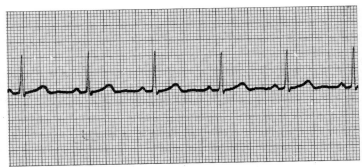

Figure 2–13. Normal sinus rhythm.

QRS Complex. This is usually normal, 0.08 to 0.11 second.

P Wave. This is upright in Lead I and II and is negative in AVR. Normal contour.

P-QRS Relationship. There is one P wave per one QRS complex; P precedes QRS with a P-R interval of normal and constant duration, 0.12 to 0.20.

Origin

NSR originates in the sinus node.

Significance

NSR indicates that electrical conduction is normal.

CARDIAC MONITOR

Definition

A cardiac monitor is a single-channel ECG apparatus with a bedside oscilloscope that allows for continuous surveillance of cardiac rhythm. The power source (battery pack) may be portable (e.g., telemetry) or stationary.

Lead Variations

The lead to be used is determined by electrode placement or a lead selector switch. Any chest or limb lead may be used. The lead chosen depends upon unit preference or what aspect of the ECG pattern is under surveillance. The most commonly used monitoring leads and some of the particular diagnostic advantages of each are listed as follows.

1. Lead II.
   a. Good P wave and QRS complex visibility (P wave is usually largest in this lead).
   b. All complexes are usually of good height and positive polarity.
2. MCL_1 (modified V_1): Its positive (+) electrode is placed at V_1 position and its negative (−) electrode is placed at the upper left chest.
   a. Determination of aberrancy or aberration versus ventricular ectopy.
   b. Differentiation of right and left premature ventricular contractions (PVCs).
   c. Determination of shift in electrode site of pacing catheter.
   d. Identification of RBBB and LBBB.
3. MCL_6 (modified V_6): Its positive electrode is placed at V_6 position and its negative electrode is placed at the upper left chest.
   a. Tall, positive QRS complexes.
   b. Detection of ST segment, T wave changes.
   c. Identification of RBBB.
   d. Identification of left ventricular (LV) ectopy.

Indications

1. Continuous identification or interpretation of cardiac rhythms or dysrhythmias.
2. Calculation of heart rate.

Limitations

Cardiac monitoring cannot accurately diagnose myocardial infarction, chamber enlargement or axis deviation.

NURSING IMPLICATIONS

Related to ECG Recording

1. A quality ECG recording should be obtained for easy and accurate interpretation.
2. A well-recorded ECG should have
   a. Correct standardization of voltage (1 mv = 1 cm).
   b. Sharp and stable baseline.
   c. Clear, exact and complete waves or complexes.

3. Have the patient lie in a comfortable position, if possible, to eliminate or avoid muscle motion and twitching.
4. Obtain proper contact between the skin and electrode. The skin should be shaved, and excessive body oil should be wiped off with alcohol.
5. Correctly place the electrodes of the precordial leads.
6. Properly ground the machine as well as the patient in order to avoid alternating current interference.

Related to Continuous Cardiac Monitoring

1. The noted arrhythmias should always be correlated with the patient's clinical status. Interference may mimic ventricular fibrillation on the oscilloscope.
2. Interference, making arrhythmia interpretation exceedingly difficult, may be caused by improper electrode placement, improper electrode application, a loose lead, patient movement (including tremors or toothbrushing), damaged equipment or improper grounding.
3. Proper selection and preparation of the electrode site aids in the assurance of a quality ECG tracing. This may be accomplished by avoiding placement on skeletal muscle, shaving the chosen area and cleansing with alcohol.
4. Electrodes should be changed daily, and the area should be cleansed. If the patient complains of "itching" or discomfort at the electrode site, skin irritation may have developed. The electrode should be removed, the site should be cleansed, and the electrode should be reapplied in a new area.
5. A false monitor display of increased heart rate will occur if the machine's sensitivity is set too high or a lead is chosen in which the P waves or T waves are as tall as the QRS complexes.
6. A false monitor display of decreased heart rate will occur if the machine's sensitivity is set too low or a lead is chosen in which the QRS complexes are almost isoelectric.
7. Explain to the patient the purpose of the cardiac monitor and assure him or her that it has no control over the heart beat.

SUGGESTED READINGS

Friedman, H. H.: *Diagnostic Electrocardiography and Vectorcardiography.* New York, McGraw-Hill, 1977.

Goldman, M. J.: *Principles of Clinical Electrocardiography*, 10th ed. Los Altos, Lange Medical Publications, 1979.

Marriott, H. J.: *Practical Electrocardiography*, 6th ed. Baltimore, Williams and Williams, 1977.

Marriott, H. J.: *Workshop in Electrocardiography*. Oldsmar, Florida, Tampa Tracings, 1975.

Millar, S. (ed.): *Methods in Critical Care*. Philadelphia, W. B. Saunders, 1980.

3

CARDIAC ENZYMES

DEFINITION

Enzymes

These are proteins that catalyze chemical reactions. Organ-specific enzymes are a form of non–plasma-specific enzymes that exist in high concentrations in the cells of various organs and skeletal muscle and are normally present in the plasma in small amounts. Cardiac enzymes are organ-specific enzymes that are present in high concentrations in myocardial tissue.

Isoenzymes

These are different molecular forms of an enzyme. The parts or subunits of an enzyme can be separated by electrophoresis. Each isoenzyme is specific for one particular organ tissue; therefore, electrophoretic separation can isolate the organ responsible for the total enzyme elevation. Both creatine phosphokinase (CPK) and lactate dehydrogenase (LDH) have subunits specific for the heart.

RATIONALE

Tissue damage can release enzymes from their intracellular storage areas. Myocardial infarction causes cellular anoxia, which alters membrane permeability and allows leakage of cellular contents. Prolonged anoxia leads to cellular edema and rupture, with consequent spillage of enzymes into surrounding tissue. Enzymes are liberated into the blood stream via the coronary lymphatic drainage system. Plasma uptake of these enzymes can be detected by serial assays, which demonstrate the rising plasma concentrations.

TYPES OF CARDIAC ENZYMES

The various cardiac enzymes peak at different times and levels (See Table 3–1). The normal values for the enzymes

Table 3–1. CARDIAC ENZYMES

ENZYME	POSITIVE FINDINGS	RISES	PEAKS	RETURNS TO NORMAL	OTHER CAUSES OF ELEVATION
CPK	5 to 10 times normal	4 to 8 hours	18 to 30 hours	3 to 4 days; *usually* in 60 to 72 hours	Muscular or neuromuscular disease Vigorous exercise IM injections Trauma or surgery
CPK-MB	MB fraction greater than 5 per cent of total CPK	2 to 4 hours	24 to 36 hours	Disappears within 30 to 72 hours; *usually* 48 hours	Crescendo angina or coronary insufficiency causing myocardial ischemia
SGOT	2 to 3 times normal	4 to 6 hours	24 to 36 hours	4 to 7 days	Polymyositis Congestive heart failure Hepatic congestion Liver disease Prolonged tachycardia Myocarditis Muscle injury
LDH	2 to 3 times normal	8 to 24 hours	2 to 5 days	Usually in 8 to 9 days; may persist 10 days to 2 weeks	Hemolysis of specimen Liver disease Anemia Pulmonary infarction Malignant tumor Skeletal muscle disease
LDH isoenzyme	LDH[1] greater than LDH[2] (flipped pattern)	12 to 24 hours	12 to 48 hours	3 to 5 days	Hemolysis of specimen Renal infarction Hemolysis due to valve prosthesis

depend on the laboratory methods used to assay them and, therefore, may vary from hospital to hospital. Five enzyme tests are commonly available.

Creatine Phosphokinase (CPK or CK)

This is the first enzyme to increase after myocardial infarction (MI). CPK is found in the heart, skeletal muscle and brain. The CPK serum level is normally higher in men than in women and is greater in persons with a large skeletal muscle mass or in those who are physically active.

CPK Isoenzymes (CPK-MB or CK II or CK-MB)

This is one of the three subunits, or bands, of CPK. The MM band is from skeletal muscle, BB is from the brain and MB is from the myocardium. The presence of the MB band with a greater quantity than 5 per cent of total CPK or greater than 10 International Units signifies myocardial damage.

Serum Glutamic Oxaloacetic Transaminase (SGOT)

This enzyme, also known as serum aspartate aminotransferase (SAPT), rises more slowly than CPK after myocardial infarction. It is widely distributed in tissues, especially the heart, liver, skeletal muscle, kidney, pancreas, spleen, lungs and red blood cells. The low specificity of this enzyme has caused this test to be used less frequently.

Lactate Dehydrogenase (LDH)

This is the last cardiac enzyme whose levels rise after infarction. It is found in the heart, kidney, skeletal muscle, liver, spleen, pancreas and red blood cells.

LDH Isoenzyme (LDH^1)

LDH^1 is specific for the heart, kidney and red blood cells. LDH has five isoenzymes, which are normally present in the serum in fixed ratios. The LDH^2 isoenzyme is usually present in the serum in greater concentration than LDH^1. If the ratio becomes reversed, or "flipped," and LDH^1 is greater than LDH^2, it is usually due to myocardial cell necrosis and indicates myocardial infarction. The flipped pattern occurs in

80 per cent of myocardial infarction patients within 1 to 3 days following MI.

INDICATIONS

Diagnosis of MI

Almost 75 per cent of patients with myocardial infarction can be diagnosed by electrocardiogram and clinical features. In these cases, elevated enzyme levels merely confirm the diagnosis. When the clinical picture is less characteristic and the electrocardiogram is normal or has nonspecific changes, verification may rely on enzyme evaluation. Positive findings of both CPK-MB and flipped LDH isoenzymes are considered 100 per cent indicative of MI.

Estimation of Myocardial Damage

When patients with acute MI have elevations of enzyme levels 8 to 10 times the normal level, inhospital mortality rises markedly. These patients have increased incidence of serious arrhythmias, congestive heart failure and cardiogenic shock.

NURSING CONSIDERATIONS

1. The purpose of drawing cardiac enzymes should be explained to the patient to increase his or her understanding of the process of diagnosis and decrease resentment at the discomfort and frequency of the procedure.
2. Intramuscular injections can cause an elevation of the CPK level and, therefore, should be avoided in persons suspected of myocardial infarction.
3. It is important to be aware of events that contribute to enzyme elevation and false labeling of major necrosis. Cardiopulmonary resuscitation (CPR), defibrillation, various diseases and trauma may make it difficult to assess "pure" serum enzyme elevations.
4. Blood specimens should be transferred to the laboratory as soon as possible to avoid hemolysis and false assays.
5. Time schedules for draws should optimize the detection of peak levels of various enzymes, as listed in Table 3–1. Patients who have had pain for several hours or even days at home are suspect for older infarctions, and assays should

be adjusted accordingly. In addition, larger MIs may peak later, as the large area of myocardial necrosis and coagulopathy may delay enzyme leakage through the swollen, thickened tissue.

6. Recurrence of chest pain during the rehabilitation phase of hospitalization may indicate extension or reinfarction and warrants enzyme re-evaluation.

SUGGESTED READINGS

Frohlich, J., Brosseuk, A., Grant, A., and Mc Lennan, M.: Study of the value of CPK and LDH isoenzyme determinations in the differential diagnosis of ischemic chest pain. *Clin. Biochem.*, 11:232–234, 1978.

Ruff, W. L., Worrell, R., and Ng, K.: Diagnostic value of creatine phosphokinase (CPK) isoenzymes in the absence of elevated total CPK. *J. Nat. Med. Assoc.*, 71:383–386, 1979.

Scheer, E.: Enzymatic changes and myocardial infarction: A nursing approach. *Cardiovasc. Nurs.*, 14:5–8, 1978.

Sher, P. P.: Cardiac isoenzymes: Better tests for diagnosing myocardial infarction. *Consultant*, October 1978, 18:166–170.

Tiongson, J. G., Jr., and Woods, A. L.: Cardiac isoenzymes: Clinical implications and limitations. *Crit. Care Q.*, 2:47–51, 1979.

Walter, P. F.: Enzymes in recognition and management of coronary syndromes. *CVP*, July-August 1976, 4:33–41.

4

FLUID AND ELECTROLYTES

GENERAL CONSIDERATIONS

The elaborate and delicate balance of body fluid and electrolytes provides an internal milieu vital for survival. The cardiovascular system is greatly affected by this balance, any alteration of which can produce mechanical and electrical myocardial disturbances. Conversely, cardiovascular disorders may negatively influence fluid and electrolyte regulation. Routine admission laboratory work for the cardiac patient should include an electrolyte profile. In addition, daily weights, intake and output should be measured on all cardiac patients, as their condition allows. To assess and anticipate accurately the physiological needs of these patients, it is extremely useful for the coronary care nurse to possess a basic understanding of the dynamics of fluid and electrolyte equilibrium.

FLUIDS

Body Fluid Disturbances

1. Total body water (TBW) is distributed proportionately between two fluid compartments: extracellular fluid (ECF) and intracellular fluid (ICF). The ECF is made up of approximately one third of the TBW, whereas the ICF constitutes two thirds. The ECF can be further subdivided into interstitial fluid and plasma.
2. Total body water represents approximately 60 per cent of the total body weight. The distribution of the TBW can be broken down as follows:

TBW of a 75 kg male = 45 kg (60%) = 45 liters

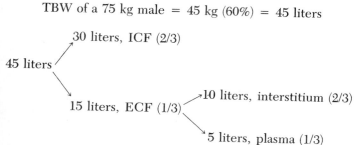

3. The major electrolytes in the ECF are sodium, chloride, bicarbonate and protein. The major ICF electrolytes include potassium, magnesium, phosphate and protein.

Terms Related to Fluid Balance

Osmolality. This refers to the total number of dissolved particles (solute) per liter of solvent (water). Serum osmolality is 300 mOsm per liter (approximately two times the serum sodium level + 10). Osmolality controls the movement and distribution of water between and within body fluid compartments. Water always moves from areas of lower osmolality (solute concentration) to areas of higher osmolality.

Hyperosmolality (Hypertonicity). This expresses an increase in solute relative to water or a decrease in water relative to solute.

Hypo-osmolality (Hypotonicity). This expresses a decrease in solute relative to water or an increase in water relative to solute.

Iso-osmolality (Isotonicity). This reflects the same solute concentration (osmolality) as plasma.

Hydrostatic Pressure. This refers to the pressure of blood cells and plasma within the capillaries, which acts to force water out of the vessels. This pressure is dependent upon (1) arterial blood pressure, (2) venous pressure, and (3) rate of blood flow through the capillaries. Normal hydrostatic pres-

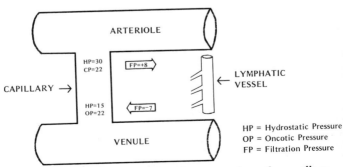

Figure 4–1. Filtration and reabsorption along the capillary.

Table 4–1. BODY FLUID IMBALANCES

	ECF EXCESS (SALINE EXCESS, HYPERVOLEMIA)	ECF DEFICIT (SALINE DEPLETION, HYPOVOLEMIA)	ICF EXCESS (WATER EXCESS, HYPONATREMIA)	ICF DEFICIT (WATER DEPLETION, HYPERNATREMIA)
Etiology	Renal, liver and heart failure with kidney retention of Na^+ and H_2O. Steroid therapy; hypoproteinemia	Vomiting Nasogastric suctioning Diarrhea Profuse diaphoresis Third spacing (burns, ascites) Adrenal insufficiency	Saline depletion with only H_2O replacement Severe renal and heart failure Inappropriate ADH secretion (stress)	Osmotic diuresis (mannitol, diabetes mellitus) Inability to respond to thirst Hyperaldosteronism Diabetes insipidus
Signs and symptoms	Normal serum Na^+ Weight gain Edema Rales ↑ Jugular veins	Normal serum Na^+ Weight loss (unless third spacing) Orthostatic hypotension Oliguria	Serum Na^+ <130 mEq/liter Normal hematocrit CNS dysfunction: confusion, stupor, headache,	Serum Na^+ >145 mEq/liter Normal hematocrit Doughy skin Thirst

↑ Central venous pressure (CVP) ↑ Pulmonary artery wedge pressure (PAWP)	Poor skin turgor Dry mucous membranes Thirst ↑ Hematocrit ↓ CVP, ↓ PAWP	coma, seizures Anorexia Nausea and vomiting ↓ Urinary specific gravity	Cell swelling; CNS irritability (due to brain cell shrinkage): confusion, stupor, muscle twitching, headache, coma, seizure ↑ Urinary specific gravity
Treatment	Diuretics Na^+ and fluid restriction	Replace saline with isotonic NaCl (IV or PO). Treat underlying cause.	Restrict free water intake.	Give free water PO or IV (D_5W)
Special considerations	May be concurrent with ICF excess (i.e., congestive heart failure) and require water restriction as well. Take daily weights.	Provide juices and broth to quench thirst (avoid excess water intake). Caution patient about arising slowly from a reclining position (orthostatic hypotension).	Often concurrent with ECF deficit, so may need to replace saline.	Caution with rapid H_2O replacement; monitor cardiovascular and CNS status during treatment.

sure ranges from 25 to 30 mm Hg at the arteriolar end and 10 to 15 mg Hg at the venular end.

Colloid Osmotic Pressure (Oncotic Pressure).   This refers to the pressure exerted by plasma proteins, which acts to hold water within the vessels or attract water that has escaped the vessels. Normal oncotic pressure is 22 to 25 mm Hg.

Filtration Pressure.   This is the result of hydrostatic pressure minus colloid pressure; it determines water movements in or out of the capillaries. (See Figure 4–1.)

Disorders of Body Fluid Balance

These can be conceptualized as saline (ECF) and water (ICF) imbalances. (See Table 4–1.)

1. *Disorders of water (ICF) balance* are reflected by changes in body osmolality. Water excess or deficit occurs when
   a. There is a ↓ or ↑ in body solute with no change in body water.
   b. There is a ↑ or ↓ in body water with no change in body solute.
   c. When a water deficit is suspected (osmolality > 300 mOsm per liter), the amount of deficit can be calculated and necessary replacement estimated.

$$\text{Normal TBW (in liters)} \doteq (0.6) \times (\text{weight in kg})$$

$$\text{Abnormal TBW (in liters)} = \frac{(\text{normal serum Na}^+)\,(\text{normal TBW})}{\text{Observed serum Na}^+}$$

$$\text{Water deficit} = \text{normal TBW} - \text{abnormal TBW}$$

For example, for a 60-kg individual with a serum Na^+ level of 160 mEq per liter,

$$\text{Normal TBW} = (0.6) \times (60 \text{ kg}) = 36 \text{ liters}$$

$$\text{Abnormal TBW} = \frac{(140)\,(36)}{(160)} = 31.5 \text{ liters}$$

The water deficit = 36 liters − 31.5 liters = 4.5 liters

Table 4–2. APPROXIMATE COMPOSITION OF BODY FLUIDS

BODY FLUID	Na⁺ (mEq/liter)	K⁺ (mEq/liter)	Cl⁻ (mEq/liter)	H⁺ (mEq/liter)	HCO₃⁻ (mEq/liter)	TONICITY	VOLUME ml/24 hours
Sweat	50	5	55	90	0	Hypotonic	Varied
Saliva	15	30	15	Varies	50–90	Hypotonic	1500
Gastric	40–80	10	140	90	0	Hypotonic	2500
Bile	135	10	105	0	35	Isotonic	500
Pancreatic	135	5	50	0	90	Isotonic	700
Small intestine	130	10	100	0	30	Isotonic	3000
Diarrhea	100	35	90	0	45	Hypotonic	500–17,000
Urine	50	40	90	Varies	Varies	Depends on excreted solute	500–12,000

2. *Saline (ECF) balance* is dependent upon a balance between the interstitial and intravascular compartments. This
   is affected by
   a. Hydrostatic pressure within the vascular bed.
   b. Oncotic pressure (protein content of plasma).
   c. Integrity of the vascular walls (keeping protein within
      the vascular compartment).

ELECTROLYTES

General Descriptions

1. Electrolytes are chemical compounds with relatively unstable electrovalent bonds. When dissolved in H_2O, they
   tend to dissociate (ionize) into electrically charged particles
   (ions). Postively charged $(+)$ ions are called cations. Negatively charged $(-)$ ions are anions. Common body cations
   include sodium (Na^+), potassium (K^+), calcium (Ca^{++}) and
   magnesium (Mg^{++}). Principal body anions are chloride
   (Cl^-), bicarbonate (HCO_3^-) and phosphate $(PO_4^{\equiv})$. Other
   anions include a few nondiffusible intracellular proteins.
   Electrolytes may be lost through various body fluids. The
   amount and distribution are listed in Table 4–2.
2. Electrolytes perform many essential physiological functions: maintaining intra- and extracellular metabolism,
   acid-base balance and neuromuscular activities.

Terms Related to Electrolyte Balance

Millimol (mM).   A mol is the molecular weight of a substance
in grams. A millimol, therefore, is 1/1000 mol.

Milliequivalent (mEq).   This measures the chemical activity
or combining power of an ion. It is mathematically derived
in the following manner:

$$\frac{\text{Mol weight (gm)}}{\text{Valence (of the substance)} \times 1000}$$

Electrolyte abnormalities are outlined in Tables 4–3 to 4–
6. The compositions of common intravenous solutions are
given in Table 4–7.

Table 4–3. SODIUM (Na$^+$)*

HYPERNATREMIA (Water Deficit)	HYPONATREMIA (Water Excess)
Definition Serum Na$^+$ >145 mEq/liter	*Definition* Serum Na$^+$ <135 mEq/liter
Etiology 1. ↑ *Water loss* Osmotic diuresis (mannitol, hyperglycemia) Diabetes insipidus Diarrhea without water replacement Renal disease	*Etiology* 1. ↑ *Water gain* Saline depletion with excessive water replacement Increased ADH stimulation (i.e., stress, ↑ intracranial pressure) Psychogenic polydipsia Adrenal insufficiency Iatrogenic infusion of excess water
2. ↑ *Body solute* Inability to drink water (coma, unavailability) Hyperaldosteronism Concentrated tube feeding Hyperalimentation	2. ↑ *Na$^+$ loss* Diuretics Salt-wasting renal disease Diarrhea, vomiting diaphoresis with only water replacement
Signs and symptoms Thirst, oliguria, confusion, lethargy, irritability, headache, convulsions, ↑ urinary specific gravity	*Signs and symptoms* Fatigue, nausea, vomiting, confusion, muscle twitching, convulsions, coma, ↓ urinary specific gravity
Management 1. Careful replacement of free water PO or IV (D$_5$W), monitoring CNS status throughout. 2. Monitor vital signs, intake and output, daily weights, serum Na$^+$ and urine. Urinary specific gravity measured during replacement. 3. Have water readily available for immobile patients.	*Management* 1. Restrict free water intake. 2. Treat cause (i.e., saline replacement, cortisone treatment). 3. Monitor intake and output, daily weights and serum Na$^+$ during management. 4. Prevent by avoiding excessive use of hypotonic irrigation solutions. 5. Teach patients to respond to thirst by drinking soups and juices.

*Normal values: 135–145 mEq per liter.
Correction: Serum osmolality (approximately two times the serum Na$^+$ plus 10) increases 5.6 mEq per liter for every 100 mg per deciliter increase over normal in blood glucose levels.

Table 4–4.   POTASSIUM (K⁺)*

HYPERKALEMIA	HYPOKALEMIA

Definition
  Serum K^+ >5.5 mEq/liter
Etiology
1. Acidosis (K^+ "shifts" out of cell as H^+ moves into cell).
2. Renal failure.
3. Severe muscle trauma, burns, ischemia.
4. Adrenal insufficiency.
5. Excessive K^+ intake (PO or IV).
6. Transfusions of banked blood.
7. False-positive findings from hemolysed blood sample.
Signs and symptoms
1. Nausea, diarrhea, cramps, muscle weakness, flaccid paralysis.
2. ECG changes: high, peaked T waves and depressed ST segments, disappearance of P waves and widening QRS complex, cardiac arrhythmias.
	Definition
	  Serum K^+ <3.5 mEq/liter
	Etiology
	1. Vomiting, diarrhea, laxative abuse, nasogastric suctioning.
	2. Alkalosis (K^+ moves into cells as H^+ moves out).
	3. Profuse wound exudate and diaphoresis.
	4. Diuretics.
	5. Potassium-poor diets.
	6. Hyperaldosteronism.
	
	Signs and symptoms
	1. Muscular weakness (primarily lower extremities), lethargy, hyporeflexia, flaccid paralysis, paralytic ileus, digitalis hypersensitivity.
	2. ECG changes: flat or inverted T waves, depression of ST segments, U waves present (especially V_2, V_3), ventricular arrhythmias.

HYPERKALEMIA	**HYPOKALEMIA**

10.0 mEq/l ——————————————————————   —————————————————— 2.5 mEq/l

Table 4–4. **POTASSIUM (K⁺)*** *Continued*

HYPERKALEMIA	HYPOKALEMIA
Management: The following may be used depending on the severity of the hyperkalemia.	*Management*
1. Glucose and insulin: 250 ml of 20% glucose with 20 to 30 units of regular insulin given IV over 20 to 30 minutes.	1. Careful K^+ replacement giving KCl orally or IV. IV replacement should not exceed 240 mEq/24 hours. In emergencies, 40 mEq/hour can be given if sufficiently diluted.
2. $NaHCO_3$: 1 to 2 amps IV push. Effect is immediate and lasts 30 to 60 minutes.	2. Instruction of diet and K^+ supplementation to patients receiving diuretics and concurrent digitalis. Foods high in K^+ include dried peaches, bananas, maple syrup, oranges, prunes, salt substitute.
3. Calcium gluconate: 10 ml IV push over 2 to 3 minutes. Repeat q 5 to 10 minutes.	
4. Kayexalate cation exchange resins (K:Na) given rectally or via nasogastric tube. Effect is delayed and should not be used in extreme emergencies.	

*Normal values: 3.5 to 5.5 mEq per liter.

Correction: A change in arterial pH by 0.1 units results in a 0.6 mEq per liter change in serum K^+ in a positive linear relationship. See nomogram in Appendix 2–7.

Table 4–5.   CALCIUM (Ca^{++})*

HYPERCALCEMIA	HYPOCALCEMIA

Definition
Serum Ca^{++} >11 mg/dl

Etiology
1. ↑ Gastrointestinal absorption: vitamin D excess, sarcoidosis, milk-alkali syndrome.
2. ↑ Bone reabsorption: hyperparathyroidism, malignancies, immobility.
3. ↑ Free Ca^{++} in blood: acidosis, adrenal insufficiency, phosphate depletion, thiazide diuretics.

Signs and symptoms
1. Anorexia, nausea, constipation, fatigue, headache, thirst, psychosis, convulsions, polyuria, nocturia, K^{+} wasting, nephrocalcinosis.
2. Cardiac changes: short Q-T interval, AV block, tachycardia-bradycardia, hypercalcemic crisis (merging ST waves), digitalis hypersensitivity, cardiac arrest.

Management: The following may be used depending upon the etiology and severity of the hypercalcemia.
1. Rehydration with normal saline is essential. Furosemide, 40 to 80 mg IV, may increase Ca^{++} excretion.
2. Mithramycin, 25 mEq/liter in a single IV dose.
3. Inorganic phosphate, 1.5 gm (50 mM) IV over 6 to 8 hours, to promote Ca^{++} excretion (monitor serum Ca^{++} closely!)
4. Hydrocortisone, 250 mg IV every 6 to 8 hours.
5. Encourage mobility or at least passive exercise.
6. Monitor intake and output and watch for saline depletion.

Definition
Serum Ca^{++} <8.0 mg/dl

Etiology
1. ↓ Gastrointestinal absorption: laxative and antacid abuse (phosphate excess), pancreatitis, malnutrition, or malabsorption.
2. ↑ Ca^{++} loss: chronic renal insufficiency, massive burns, peritonitis.
3. ↓ Free Ca^{++} in blood: alkalosis, transfusions of citrated blood, hypoparathyroidism, hypoalbuminism, hypomagnesemia.

Signs and symptoms
1. Muscle twitching, cramping, tetany, positive Chvostek's and Trousseau's sign, parathesias, grimacing, laryngospasm, carpopedal spasm.
2. Cardiac changes: prolonged Q-T interval, cardiac arrhythmia, cardiac arrest.

Management
1. Calcium gluconate (10%), 10 to 20 ml IV at 2 ml/minute.
2. Calcium drip: 15 mg Ca^{++}/kg of body weight in 1000 ml D$_5$W to run in 4 hours.
3. Counsel patient regarding calcium intake in diet and misuse of antacids and laxatives.
4. Maintain seizure precautions until Ca^{++} levels return to normal.

---

*Normal values: 8.8 to 10.4 mg per deciliter or 4.5 to 5.5 mEq per liter.
Correction: Add 0.8 mg per deciliter to Ca^{++} value for every *decrease* in serum albumin by 1 gm per deciliter (normal = 3.5 to 5.2 gm per deciliter). This calculation is reversed for elevated albumin levels.

Table 4–6. MAGNESIUM (Mg^{++})*

HYPERMAGNESEMIA	HYPOMAGNESEMIA

Definition
   Serum Mg^{++} >2.5 mEq/liter
Etiology
1. ↑ *Mg^{++} intake*
   Hemodialysis
   Antacids and laxative misuse
   Excessive MgSO$_4$ administration
   in eclampsia
2. ↑ *Mg^{++} release from tissues*
   Catabolism
   Diabetic ketoacidosis
3. ↓ *Renal excretion*
   Adrenal insufficiency
   Chronic renal failure
Signs and symptoms
1. Weakness, paralysis, nausea,
   lethargy, confusion, respiratory
   depression, ↓ urine output.
2. Cardiac changes: slowed AV con-
   duction, hypotension, bradycar-
   dia.
	Definition
	   Serum Mg^{++} <1.5 mEq/liter
	Etiology
	1. ↑ *Loss of Mg^{++}*
	   Prolonged nasogastric suction
	   Extensive burns, diuresis
	   K$^+$ depletion, diabetic
	   ketoacidosis
	   Hypercalcemia
	2. ↓ *Intestinal Mg^{++} absorption*
	   Low intake (alcoholism)
	   Malabsorption syndrome
	   Severe diarrhea
	
	Signs and symptoms
	1. Muscle twitching, hyperreflexia,
	   positive Chvostek's and Trous-
	   seau's signs, nystagmus, insom-
	   nia.
	2. Cardiac changes: peaked T waves
	   and prolonged QRS, ventricular
	   arrhythmias; potentiates digitalis
	   effects.

Management
1. Calcium gluconate (10%), 10 to
   20 ml IV at 2 ml/minute to an-
   tagonize Mg^{++} effects.
2. Give fluids to promote increased
   urinary output.
3. Counsel patient on misuse of an-
   tacids and laxatives.
	Management
	1. Magnesium sulfate, 1 to 2 gm
	   IM or slow IV at a rate not
	   greater than 1.5 ml/minute (have
	   calcium gluconate on hand).
	2. Counsel patient on increasing
	   Mg^{++} in diet, found in whole
	   grains, meats, some fruits such
	   as bananas.

*Normal values: 1.5 to 2.5 mEq/liter.

Table 4–7. COMPOSITION OF COMMON IV SOLUTIONS

SOLUTION	TONICITY	Na$^+$ (mEq/liter)	K$^+$ (mEq/liter)	Cl$^-$ (mEq/liter)	Ca^{++} (mEq/liter)	LACTATE (mEq/liter)	DEXTROSE (gm/dl)
5% DW	Hypotonic	–	–	–	–	–	50
10% DW	Hypertonic	–	–	–	–	–	100
0.9% DW	Isotonic	154	–	–	–	–	–
5% D/0.9% NS	Isotonic	154	–	154	–	–	50
5% D/0.45% NS	Hypotonic	77	–	77	–	–	50
5% D/0.2% NS	Hypotonic	34	–	34	–	–	50
Lactated Ringer (LR)	Isotonic	130	4	109	3	28	–
LR in 5% D	Isotonic	130	4	109	3	28	50

SUGGESTED READINGS

Felver, L.: Understanding the electrolyte maze. *AJN*, 80:1591, 1980.

Rose, B.: *Clinical Physiology of Acid-Base and Electrolyte Disorders.* New York, McGraw-Hill, 1977.

Scribner, B. H. (ed.): *Teaching Syllabus for the Course on Fluid and Electrolyte Balance* 7th rev. Seattle, University of Washington, School of Medicine, 1969.

Stroot, V., et al.: *Fluid and Electrolytes.* Philadelphia, F. A. Davis, 1977.

Urrows, S.: Fluid and electrolyte balance in the patient with myocardial infarction. *Nursing Clin. North Am.*, 15:603, 1980.

5

ARTERIAL BLOOD GASES AND ACID-BASE STATUS

GENERAL CONSIDERATIONS

Assessment of oxygenation and acid-base status is indicated in nearly all acutely ill patients with cardiopulmonary disease. This provides valuable aid not only in diagnosing impairments but also in guiding therapeutics. The tasks of cardiopulmonary function include oxygen uptake in the lungs, oxygen–carbon dioxide exchange in the tissues and carbon dioxide transport to the lungs for elimination. Cardiovascular impairment, as seen in cardiogenic shock, impedes task fulfillment. The result is inadequate tissue perfusion with excessive anaerobic metabolism and lactic acid accumulation. In addition, cardiovascular performance is extremely sensitive to changes in the chemical milieu and suffers with even small changes in hydrogen ion (H^+) concentration or decreases in the oxygen supply. Clinical signs and symptoms are not sufficient to detect acid-base derangements. The only reliable method is measurement of blood pH.

DEFINITIONS

pH (7.35–7.45)

The pH expresses the acid-base status of the body in terms of H^+ concentration (pH $= -$ log $[H^+]$). At a normal blood pH of 7.40, the H^+ concentration is 0.00004 mEq per liter. Any pH values of less then 6.8 or greater than 7.8 prove fatal, as vital enzymes fail to function in these environments.

Po_2 (80–100 mm Hg)

This value measures the partial pressure of oxygen dissolved in 100 ml of plasma. Po_2 usually decreases with age.

Pco_2 (35–45 mm Hg)

This value measures the partial pressure of carbon dioxide dissolved in 100 ml of plasma. It is regulated by alveolar ventilation; thus, it represents respiratory acid-base status.

Oxygen Saturation (80–100 Per Cent)

This value expresses the ratio between the oxygen-carrying capacity of the red blood cells (hemoglobin [Hb]) and the amount of oxygen they are actually carrying.

$$\frac{O_2 \text{ combined with Hb}}{O_2 \text{ capacity of Hb}}$$

HCO_3^- (22–25 mEq)

This value measures the free bicarbonate ion present in the blood and represents the renal-regulated (metabolic) portion of the body's acid-base status.

Total CO_2 Content (25–27 mEq/liter)

This value is a direct measurement of all CO_2 dissolved in the blood. CO_2 is found in three major forms: bicarbonate ion (HCO_3^-), carbonic acid (H_2CO_3) and dissolved gas (PCO_2). As the latter two forms account for a relatively small amount of total CO_2, this value is representative of HCO_3^- concentration.

Acidosis

Acidosis is a process resulting in either increased acid or decreased base, reflecting a high H^+ concentration and a low blood pH.

Alkalosis

Alkalosis is a process resulting in either increased base or decreased acid, reflecting a low H^+ concentration and a high blood pH.

RATIONALE

Acid-Base Regulation

The body strives to keep the blood pH between 7.35 and 7.45. To do so, it must maintain a 20 to 1 ratio between bicarbonate ion and carbonic acid (Fig. 5–1). Four regulatory systems aid in the body's defense against pH changes.

Chemical Buffers. These provide the fastest response to changes in H^+ concentration. Hemoglobin works rapidly,

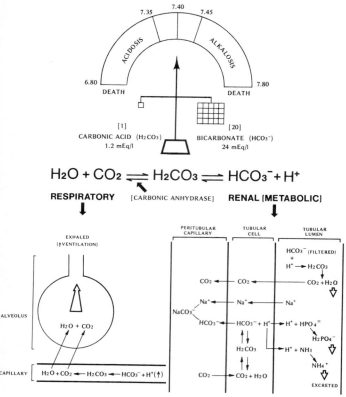

Figure 5–1. Acid-base regulation.

combining with H^+ as HCO_3^- moves out of the cell into the extracellular fluid.

Lungs. These organs are the body's next line of defense. By altering rate and depth of respirations, H^+ in the form of carbonic acid is reduced to CO_2 and H_2O, both of which are exhaled.

The Cells. These provide assistance within 1 to 4 hours. As pH falls, H^+ diffuses into the cells and combines with a conjugate base. To maintain electroneutrality, potassium (K^+) moves out of the cells, raising serum K^+. An inward flux of K^+ occurs as pH rises.

The Kidneys. These organs work slowly (in 1 to 4 days) to maintain H^+ homeostasis. This is done through HCO_3^- reabsorption and H^+ secretion by the proximal and distal renal tubule cells.

Compensation. Compensation for acid-base imbalances occurs when the system (respiratory or metabolic) not primarily affected is responsible for returning blood pH to normal. The body *does not overcompensate.*

Oxygenation

Hemoglobin has an affinity for oxygen and combines reversibly with it. Fully saturated, 1 gm of hemoglobin carries 1.34 ml of oxygen. As normal hemoglobin concentration is 15 gm per deciliter of blood, the oxygen-carrying capacity of the blood is 20 ml per deciliter of blood. The affinity of hemoglobin for oxygen depends critically upon the partial pressure of oxygen (PO_2). Cyanosis occurs when hemoglobin is reduced (desaturated) by at least 5 gm per deciliter of blood. Severely

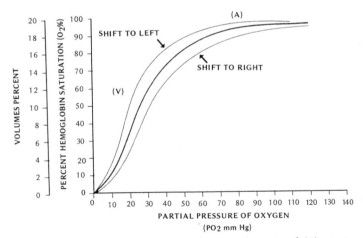

Figure 5–2. Oxyhemoglobin curve. The flat arterial (A) portion of the curve reflects little change in oxyhemoglobin saturation with a large change in oxygen tension (Po_2). The venous (V) portion implies a very loose oxygen affinity with great changes in oxyhemoglobin saturation for a very small change in Po_2. A rightward shift of the curve reflects decreased hemoglobin affinity for oxygen and occurs with ↓ pH, ↑ Pco_2, ↑ temperature and ↑ DPG; a leftward shift implies a greater oxygen affinity and occurs with ↑ pH, ↓ Pco_2, ↓ temperature and ↓ DPG.

Table 5–1. ACID-BASE DISORDERS

	RESPIRATORY ACIDOSIS	RESPIRATORY ALKALOSIS	METABOLIC ACIDOSIS	METABOLIC ALKALOSIS
Definition	Reduced alveolar ventilation relative to the rate of carbon dioxide production, resulting in increased carbonic acid	Increased alveolar ventilation relative to the rate of carbon dioxide production	Physiologic process characterized by: the primary *gain of* H^+ or primary *loss of* HCO_3^-	Primary *gain of* HCO_3^- or *loss of* H^+ by the extracellular fluid
Findings	pH $\downarrow$ P_{CO_2} $\uparrow$ HCO_3^- normal ($\uparrow$ with compensation)	pH $\uparrow$ P_{CO_2} $\downarrow$ HCO_3^- normal ($\downarrow$ with compensation)	pH $\downarrow$ P_{CO_2} normal ($\downarrow$ with compensation) HCO_3^- $\downarrow$	pH $\uparrow$ P_{CO_2} normal ($\uparrow$ with compensation) HCO_3^- $\uparrow$
Causes	Obstructive lung disease Oversedation Pickwickian syndrome Airway obstruction Neuromuscular disorders Hypoventilation	Hypoxia Psychogenic hyperventilation Salicylate overdose (initial) Congestive heart failure Hepatic coma Fever Brain lesions	*Gain of* H^+ ($\uparrow$ anion gap) Diabetic ketoacidosis Poisoning: Salicylate Ethylene glycol Methyl alcohol Paraldehyde Lactic acidosis Renal failure	Diuretic therapy Vomiting, nasogastric drainage Corticosteroids Cushing's syndrome (aldosteronism) Banked blood transfusions Overtreatment with $NaHCO_3$

			Loss of HCO_3^- (normal anion gap) Diarrhea Drainage of pancreatic juice Acetazolamide (Diamox) treatment Renal tubular disease	
Signs and Symptoms	Headache, tremor, confusion, lethargy, coma, arrhythmia	Numbness and tingling of extremities, carpalpedal spasms, vertigo, arrhythmia	Hypotension, nausea, vomiting, lethargy, coma, Kussmaul's breathing (ketoacidosis), arrhythmia	Nausea, vomiting, diarrhea, sensorium changes, tremors, convulsions, arrhythmia
Management	Treat underlying cause. Increase the depth and rate of ventilation.	Treat underlying cause. Rebreathing bag or sedation is used to treat psychogenic hyperventilation.	Treat underlying cause. If pH is 7.2, $NaHCO_3$ should be given. (Dose = weight in kg × deficiency of HCO_3 × 0.3) Give one third of calculated dose and recheck blood gases.	Treat the underlying cause. K^+ depletion may be the cause of consequence of this process and may require replacement in the form of KCL.

anemic patients may never develop cyanosis, whereas patients with polycythemia may become very cyanotic with only slight decreases in PO_2. Extremely low cardiac output causes cyanosis, despite high arterial oxygen tension. The important relationship between oxygen saturation and PO_2 is demonstrated by the oxyhemoglobin curve (Fig. 5–2).

ABNORMAL FINDINGS

Acid-Base Disorders

Acid-base disorders occur secondary to a disruption in the ratio of acid to base. The four types of acid-base disturbances are described in Table 5–1.

Hypoxemia

Hypoxemia refers to an abnormally low PO_2 and is frequently associated with hypoxia or inadequate tissue oxygenation. Treatment relies on determining the cause and providing optimum ventilation and oxygenation. Hypoxemia is the result of four major problems.

Hypoventilation. This describes ventilation inadequate to meet metabolic needs. It is always associated with a concurrent elevation in PCO_2.

Diffusion Impairment. This arises when there is an increase in the distance gas must travel from alveolus to capillary. Diffusion abnormalities result from anemia, pulmonary fibrosis, sarcoidosis and scleroderma.

Shunting. This occurs as a result of a decrease in the ventilation to perfusion ($\dot{V}/\dot{Q}$) ratio, as blood passes nonventilated alveoli. Causes include pulmonary edema, atelectasis, pneumonia and bronchial constriction.

Ventilation to Perfusion Inequality ("Dead Spacing"). This problem occurs when ventilation and blood flow are mismatched at various regions of the lung. Alveoli are underperfused secondary to impeded capillary circulation. A common cause of this is pulmonary emboli.

SUGGESTED READINGS

Lomberg, L., et al.: Arterial blood gases in the coronary care unit, Part I. *Heart and Lung*, 6:526, 1977.

Lomberg, L., et al.: Arterial blood gases in the coronary care unit, Part II. *Heart and Lung*, 6:697, 1977.

Rose, D.: *Clinical Physiology of Acid-Base and Electrolytes*. New York, McGraw-Hill, 1977.

Shapiro, B., et al.: *Clinical Application of Respiratory Care*, 2nd ed. Chicago, Year Book Medical Publishers, 1979.

Shrake, K.: The ABC's of ABG's. *Nursing '79*, 9:26, 1979.

Waldron, M.: Oxygen transport. *AJN*, 79:272, 1979.

6

COAGULATION TESTS

GENERAL CONSIDERATIONS

Coagulation

Coagulation is the process of blood clotting to maintain hemostasis. Hemostasis is prevention of blood loss.

Anticoagulant Therapy

Anticoagulant therapy involves a deliberate disruption of the natural blood-clotting mechanism. Baseline laboratory work should be performed before therapy is initiated.

Coagulation Tests

Coagulation tests evaluate the hemostatic factors and functions of the blood-clotting mechanism. They include the following:

1. Coagulation system tests, which evaluate the activities of the intrinsic and extrinsic clotting systems.
2. Platelet system tests, which screen for defects in platelet numbers and functions.

RATIONALE

Effective hemostasis is dependent on three systems: blood vessels, platelets and coagulation.

The Coagulation System

This system has two separate but interrelated clotting pathways. These are the intrinsic and extrinsic systems, which merge into the final pathway leading to fibrin formation.

Coagulation Factors (Procoagulants)

These factors participate in the clotting sequence in a cascade pattern, with each factor activating the next. Lack of any of the factors unbalances the hemostatic mechanism. Most of the procoagulants are synthesized in the liver.

INDICATIONS

Coagulation tests are utilized to

1. Diagnose hereditary hemorrhagic disorders.
2. Detect hemostatic disruption due to disease.
3. Monitor anticoagulant therapy.

TYPES OF COAGULATION TESTS

Tests of the Intrinsic Pathway

Activated Partial Thromboplastin Time (APTT). This is the time required for recalcified citrated plasma to clot. It is useful in detecting deficiencies in factors that generate thromboplastin (everything but factor X). The APTT allows assay of the factors affected by heparin. Heparin activity is monitored by measuring the APTT against a control. Normal APTT varies from laboratory to laboratory but usually is 25 to 39 seconds. Its therapeutic level is about one to one and one-half times normal.

Recalcification Time (Recal). This measure indicates the clotting time of citrated blood by recalcifying the sample with calcium chloride. The recalcification time monitors heparin therapy. The therapeutic level is two to three times baseline (normal). Normal time is 150, plus or minus 30 seconds. If intermittent therapy is used, blood should be drawn 1 hour or less prior to the next dose of heparin. The specimen must be in the lab and the test performed within 30 minutes after venipuncture.

Whole Blood Clotting Time (Coagulation Time, Lee-White Time). This is the time required for 1 ml of whole blood to clot at 37° C with controlled temperature and exposure to a glass surface. It measures the overall ability of the blood to clot. Normal clotting time varies from 7 to 15 minutes. The results are influenced by several factors, which makes consistent results difficult.

Measurement of Coagulation Factors XII, XI, IX, VIII. This is included in a study of the intrinsic system.

Tests of the Extrinsic System

Prothrombin Time or One-Stage Prothrombin Time (Pro-Time or PT). This measures the time required for recalcified plasma to clot in the presence of tissue thromboplastin. Prolonged results indicate circulating anticoagulants, a fibrinogen level below 100 mg per deciliter, or a vitamin K deficiency. A reduced pro-time may indicate multiple myeloma or thrombophlebitis. This test is used to monitor coumarin therapy. Baseline or normal time is 12 to 14 seconds. Coumarin therapeutic level is kept at 20 to 29 seconds or two to two and a half times normal. Coumarin takes 10 hours to affect coagulation, peaks in 2 to 5 days and persists 10 to 14 days after the last dose. Heparin, at the peak of its activity, will also prolong the pro-time.

Measurement of Coagulation Factors VII, II, V and X. This is included in study of the extrinsic pathway.

Tests of Platelets and Platelet Formation

Platelet Count. This measurement involves an examination of the peripheral blood smear. On a well-stained smear, there should be 8 to 12 platelets per 1000 magnification field. The normal platelet count is 150,000 to 400,000 per cubic millimeter.

Bleeding Time. This is usually normal at platelet counts of greater than 100,000 per cubic millimeter. A small lancet cut is made into the patient's finger or ear lobe, and the time required for bleeding to cease is carefully observed. Bleeding normally stops in less than 6 minutes. Extended bleeding times results from liver disease, leukemia, other bleeding disorders and excessive ingestion of aspirin.

Clot Retraction. This is a crude method of evaluating platelet and fibrinogen activity. Blood is allowed to clot in a test tube and is observed after 2 hours to see if the clot has retracted from the sides of the tube.

Other Tests

Thrombin Time (TT). This measures the time required for a standard thrombin to clot plasma. It can differentiate heparin from other anticoagulants. This detects abnormalities in the fibrinogen molecule.

Fibrinogen. This is present in measurable amounts and is reported in units of milligrams per deciliter. It should not be less than 100 mg per deciliter.

Fibrin-Fibrinogen Degradation Products (Split Fibrin, FDP or FSP). The presence of these products in abnormal amounts indicates extensive injuries or inflammatory disease. It is also the definitive test for disseminated intravascular coagulopathy.

Screening Tests

Coagulation System Tests. A commonly used set of screening tests for coagulation tests includes a prothrombin time, partial thromboplastin time, thrombin time and fibrinogen concentration.

Platelet System Tests. Basic screening includes a bleeding time and platelet count.

SUGGESTED READINGS

Byrne, J.: Hematology: coagulation studies, Part I. *Nursing '77,* 7:8, 1977.

Byrne, J.: Hematology: coagulation studies, Part II. *Nursing '77,* 7:24, June, 1977.

Hand, J.: Keeping anticoagulants under control. *R.N.,* April 1979, 42:25.

Sohn, C. A., Tannenbaum, R. P., Cantwell, R., and Rogers, M. P.: Rescinding the risks in administering anticoagulants. *Nursing '81,* 11:34, 1981.

GENERAL CONSIDERATIONS

Hemodynamic monitoring is an invasive method of continuous assessment and evaluation of pressure changes produced by blood movement throughout the cardiac cycle. It is performed at the bedside to provide information regarding the earliest changes in the circulatory system that are not always clinically detectable in the patient. However, the patient's clinical status should always be correlated with the findings of hemodynamic monitoring. Together, these data furnish guidelines for effective fluid and pharmacological management. This chapter includes discussions on monitoring of pulmonary artery pressure (PAP), cardiac output (CO), central venous pressure (CVP), and intra-arterial pressure.

PULMONARY ARTERY PRESSURE MONITORING

Definition

Pulmonary artery pressure monitoring is defined as continuous direct measurement of the pulmonary artery pressure by using a flow-directed balloon catheter.

Pulmonary Artery Pressure (PAP). This is the pressure exerted by blood against the walls of the pulmonary artery, reflecting the hemodynamics of the pulmonary vascular tree. PAP consists of the systolic, diastolic, mean PA and pulmonary artery wedge pressure (PAWP).

Pulmonary Artery Wedge Pressure (PAWP). This is a value obtained by inflating the balloon and causing it to wedge in a small branch of the pulmonary artery, thus measuring the pressure distal to the occlusion and reflecting pulmonary venous, left atrium and left ventricular pressures at the end of diastole (LVEDP). One of the major determinants of LVEDP is the end-diastolic volume of the blood (preload) in the left ventricle.

Rationale

During diastole, blood flows freely from the pulmonary arteries through the pulmonary capillaries, left atrium and

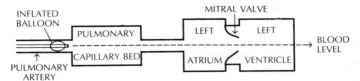

Figure 7–1. Relationship between PAWP and LVEDP. At end of diastole, PAD = PAWP = LAP = LVEDP.

open mitral valve to the left ventricle. Therefore, the pressure in the left ventricle at the end of diastole approximates the diastolic pressure in the pulmonary artery, pulmonary capillaries and left atrium. See Figure 7–1.

Procedure

Insertion. This is accomplished at the bedside via cutdown or percutaneous puncture of brachial, subclavian, jugular or femoral vein, using sterile technique. The catheter is advanced through the vein into the right atrium. The balloon is then inflated and follows the direction of the blood flow to carry the catheter through the right ventricle into the pulmonary artery, where the inflated balloon finally wedges in a right or left branch (see Fig. 7–2). The path of the balloon can be followed by wave forms seen on the pressure monitor (see Fig. 7–3).

Setup. This includes connection of the catheter to pressure tubing, continuous flushing device, transducer, pressure monitor (Fig. 7–2) and write-out machine. All tubing should be preflushed prior to connection, and the flushing system should be maintained at a pressure of 300 mm Hg by a pressurized bag.

Calibration. This is performed with the transducer at the level of the right atrium (fourth intercostal space, midaxillary line). The reference point is marked with felt pen to ensure consistency in measurement, and the pressure monitor is calibrated according to the manufacturer's specification.

Pressure Readings. These are obtained from transducer conversion of pressure to electrical signals, resulting in a digital and wave form readout. Normal pressures measured during right heart and pulmonary artery catheterization are as follows:

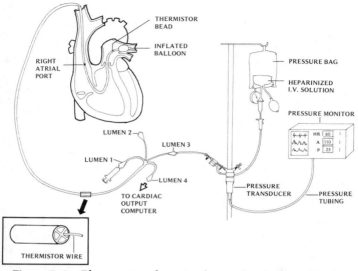

Figure 7–2. Placement and setup of a quadruple lumen pulmonary artery catheter. Lumen 1 serves for inflation of and passive deflation of the balloon. Lumen 2 terminates 30 cm from the catheter tip in the right atrium. It serves as an injector port for thermodilation cardiac output measurements and allows the measurement of right atrial pressure (CVP). Lumen 3 terminates at the tip of the catheter and allows the measurement of chamber pressures, pulmonary artery and pulmonary wedge pressures and mixed venous sampling. Lumen 4 contains two thermistor wires, which terminate in the thermistor head 4 cm from the catheter tip.

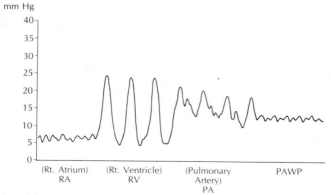

Figure 7–3. Wave forms during pulmonary arterial catheterization.

Right atrial (RA)	1–5 mm Hg
Right ventricular (RV)	25/5 mm Hg
Pulmonary artery systolic (PAS)	25 (range, 15–30) mm Hg
Pulmonary artery diastolic (PAD)	10 (range, 5–12) mm Hg
Mean pulmonary arterial ($\overline{PA}$)	15 mm Hg
Mean pulmonary arterial wedge pressure($\overline{PAWP}$)	12 (range, 5–12) mm Hg

Therapeutic Guidelines.*   These are determined from the value of the PAWP. Abnormal findings include the following:

Onset of pulmonary congestion	18–20 mm Hg
Moderate pulmonary congestion	20–25 mm Hg
Severe pulmonary congestion	25–30 mm Hg
Onset of pulmonary edema	>30 mm Hg

In patients with pump failure, the PAWP may be maintained between 15 and 18 mm Hg to maximize left ventricular contraction according to Starling's Law. Diuretics, nitrates or cardiotonic drugs are used to lower PAWP. In patients with volume depletion, normal saline challenges may be used to increase the PAWP.

See Table 7–1 for conditions with expected pressure changes.

Indications

Moment-to-moment PA monitoring detects hemodynamic changes much earlier than clinical signs and symptoms appear. In the Coronary Care Unit, it is primarily used for assessment of left ventricular dysfunction, which may result from any of the following conditions: pump failure, hyper- or

*From Forrester, J. S., et al.: Hemodynamic therapy of myocardial infarction. N. Engl. J. Med. 295:1359, 1976.

Table 7–1. CONDITIONS WITH EXPECTED PRESSURE CHANGES

1. Normal left ventricle	Increase in LVEDP indicates an increase in blood volume. A decrease in LVEDP indicates a decrease in blood volume.
2. Heart failure or volume overload	PAP and PAWP are increased.
3. Hypovolemia	PAP and PAWP are decreased.
4. Cardiogenic shock	PAWP depends on the ability of the failing heart to handle the circulating volume.
5. Mitral valve disease	Unreliable pressure readings are obtained in this disease.
6. Pulmonary hypertension	PA is increased. PAWP may or may not be increased.
7. Pulmonary emboli	Usually PA is increased and PAWP is decreased.

hypovolemia, shock, pulmonary hypertension or pulmonary emboli.

Complications

Invasive procedures always carry some risk. Reported PAP monitoring complications include

1. Pneumothorax and arrhythmias during insertion.
2. Pulmonary artery perforation.
3. Pulmonary infarction.
4. Thrombophlebitis at the cutdown site.
5. Pulmonary embolism.
6. Sepsis or infection.
7. Air embolism.

Nursing Management

Preprocedure

a. Explain the purpose and general procedure of insertion. Assure the patient that there is minimal discomfort, although he or she may feel the tube passing through the vein. Stress the importance of not moving during the procedure. Help the patient into a comfortable position.
b. Obtain written permission.
c. Assemble necessary equipment and the supplies, including the crash cart, as specified by hospital policies.
d. Prepare and calibrate the pressure monitor, as stated earlier.

During Procedure

Stay close to and reassure the patient. Check vital signs frequently. Observe cardiac monitor for the presence of arrhythmias. Read and record RA, RV, PA pressures and PAWP. Upon completion of the insertion, apply a dry sterile dressing to the insertion site. Elastoplast tape is used to prevent oozing and to secure the catheter in place.

Postprocedure

Monitor and Record PA Pressures. This should be performed hourly or as indicated. The monitor should be calibrated every 4 hours or as specified by the manufacturer to correct for electronic drift. The transducer should be maintained at the correct reference level with each recording. The systolic, diastolic and mean PAP can be obtained from the digital and oscilloscopic display. The PAWP is determined by injecting 0.8 to 1.5 ml of air from a syringe into the balloon port until the wedge pattern is obtained. Prolonged inflation of the balloon may result in pulmonary infarction. Deflation of the balloon is accomplished by allowing air to expel passively. Overinflation of the balloon may result in rupture; repeated inflations of a ruptured balloon can cause air emboli. Pressure readings and wave forms are recorded as indicated.

Maintain Patency of Catheter. This is accomplished by continuous flushing by the pressurized flushing device. The catheter should also be manually flushed at least every hour. Aspirate the catheter before flushing if a clot is suspected in the catheter.

Prevent Infection. Infection is prevented by using sterile technique when manipulating the catheter, dressings or pressure tubing. Change the dressing and intravenous fluid at least every 24 hours. Observe the insertion site for signs of infection.

Troubleshoot Problems. This is related to PAP monitoring. Measures used may vary according to unit policy and physicians' preference. See Table 7–2 for the commonly observed problems and alleviating measures.

Discontinue Catheter. When the continuous monitoring is no longer indicated, discontinue the use of the catheter as ordered. Catheters indwelling for longer than 3 days greatly increase the risk of infection. The catheter is removed slowly while the cardiac monitor is observed for ventricular arrhythmias. A dry sterile dressing is applied after direct pressure has been exerted over the site for 10 to 15 minutes. Check insertion site for signs of infection during the 24 hours after removal. Remove any sutures within 72 hours.

THERMODILUTION—CARDIAC OUTPUT MONITORING

Definition

Thermodilution is an indicator dilution method, using temperature change as the indicator to determine cardiac output (CO).

Rationale

A known volume of cold solution is rapidly injected into the right atrium via the proximal port of a quadruple-lumen,

Table 7–2. TROUBLESHOOTING PROBLEMS OF
PAP MONITORING

PROBLEM	INTERVENTION
I. Alteration of wave form A. Damping to disappearance of wave form	1. Turn stopcock off to the patient and flush the tubing. 2. Check for kinks, especially at the insertion site. 3. Check for air or blood in tubing. 4. Make sure all stopcocks are open to the right direction and connections are secure. 5. Ask the patient to cough in an attempt to reposition the catheter. 6. Recalibrate the pressure machine. 7. Check the transducer and change if necessary. 8. Check pressure monitor and have it repaired if necessary. 9. Consider X-ray to locate tip of catheter.
B. Continuous RV form	1. Compare wave form with previous readings. 2. Reposition the patient. 3. Inflate balloon in an attempt to flow it into the PA. 4. Consider X-ray.
C. Continuous PAWP form	1. Reposition the patient. 2. Check inflation port and make sure the balloon is deflated. 3. Pull back the catheter cautiously until disappearance of PAWP wave form if all other measures fail.
D. Fluctuation of wave form	1. This may require manipulation of the catheter. 2. Suspect catheter whip.
II. Inability to obtain PAWP	1. Check the wave form to ascertain catheter location. 2. Reposition the patient. 3. Check resistance to balloon inflation to rule out balloon rupture. 4. Inflate the balloon to advance it into a PA branch.
III. Air or blood in setup	1. Tighten all connections. 2. Aspirate from the stopcock if a clot is suspected. 3. Flush system away from the patient to clear.
IV. Increased ventricular irritability	1. Check for RV and fluctuation of wave form. Follow prestated suggestions. 2. Reposition the patient. 3. Keep antiarrhythmics within reach. Administer as indicated. 4. Be prepared to manipulate the catheter if whip is present. 5. Consider X-ray.

flow-directed pulmonary artery catheter (Fig. 7–2). The injectate then mixes with the blood. The resulting change in blood temperature is detected 26 cm (may vary according to manufacturer) downstream in the pulmonary artery by a thermistor bead located 4 cm (may vary according to manufacturer) from the catheter tip and is recorded as a time-temperature curve (Fig. 7–4). The area under this curve is calculated by an attached computer, and cardiac output is digitally displayed. The degree of temperature change is inversely proportional to the flow rate of venous blood, which approximates cardiac output. Therefore, the smaller the degree of temperature change, the larger the CO.

Procedure

1. Introduction of the thermodilution pulmonary artery catheter into the pulmonary artery is accomplished in the same manner as PA catheterization.
2. Several syringes are then filled with 5 to 10 ml of sterile injectable solution. Ten milliliters will produce a larger "signal" for the computer. Either 5 per cent dextrose and water or normal saline can be used as an injectate, depending on the patient's volume status and the unit

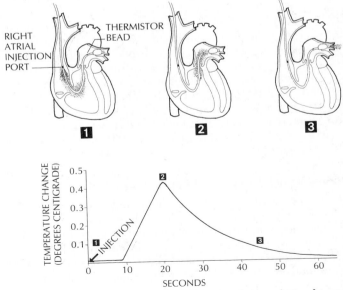

Figure 7–4. Thermodilation injection and its relationship to a time-temperature curve.

policy. The injectate may be iced (0 to 5° C) or room temperature (22 to 26° C). The latter, however, results in smaller temperature changes, which may affect accuracy in some cases. Room temperature injectates may be used in place of iced injectates if their measurements are within 10 per cent of those obtained from using iced injectates.

3. For chilled injectates, the filled syringes are placed in an icy environment using any means to ensure the sterility of injectable solution. A thermodilution temperature probe (if not built internally into the catheter) is placed in one of the filled syringes to provide an accurate temperature reading of injectate. The solution is then chilled to 0 to 5° C.

4. Calibration numbers for injectate temperature and volume should be dialed into the thermodilution computer according to computer design. Turn the computer on and wait for the ready signal. The balloon must be deflated, and the patient should be quiet during CO measurements.

5. Carefully remove a syringe from the container. Handle the syringe by the wings, avoiding the barrel to minimize rewarming of injectate. The injectate is then rapidly injected into the proximal port at a rate not slower than 10 ml in 4 seconds. A CO_2 cartridge injector gun may be used to provide fast, uniform injections. Record the CO measurement when digitally displayed. Repeat the procedure three times at 90-second intervals, preferably at the same point in this patient's respiratory cycle (i.e., end-expiration). This minimizes the effects of pulmonary artery temperature fluctuation on CO measurement.

6. Three readings are obtained, and the average is recorded. Any readings showing more than a 10 per cent variance should be deleted.

Normal Values and Clinical Application

1. Normal cardiac output in adults ranges widely from 4 to 8 liters per minute. However, these values do not take into account varied individual needs according to body size. To compensate for size differences, cardiac output indexing is often calculated. *Cardiac Index* (CI) is determined by dividing CO by body surface area (BSA).*

---

*The Dubois Body Surface Chart is in Appendix 2.

$$CI = CO/BSA$$

Example:

$$CI = \frac{CO = 6 \text{ liters/minute}}{BSA = 1.5 \text{ m}^2} = 4 \text{ liters/minute/m}^2$$

2. Serial CO measurements may be compared with serial PAWP measurements to assess ventricular function. A ventricular function curve (Frank-Starling Curve) is constructed by plotting PAWP on the horizontal (x) axis of a graph and cardiac output (or CI) on the vertical (y) axis. Such curves are constructed to guide fluid and drug therapy (see Fig. 7–5).

Indications

Thermodilution measurement is used to determine CO in a variety of situations. It may be used in shock, myocardial infarction, arrhythmia and positive end-expiratory pressure (PEEP) therapy.

Complications

1. The complications resulting from catheter insertion and placement are the same as those described for PA catheterization.

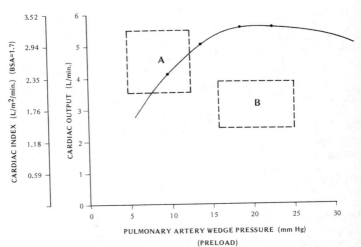

Figure 7–5. Ventricular function curve constructed by plotting results from measured CO (CI) and PAWP of a patient receiving medical therapy. *A*, Usual range in normal LV. *B*, Usual range in compromised LV.

2. Septicemia is further potentiated by the risk of injectate contamination. An iced injectate setup carries a greater risk than a room temperature setup.
3. Volume overload may result from too frequent cardiac output determinations, particularly with use of 10-ml volumes.
4. Air embolization can occur secondary to air in the injectate.
5. Ventricular arrhythmias may occur (rarely) following injection of the cold indicator.

Nursing Management

1. Explain the general procedure and purpose of thermodilution cardiac output measurements to the patient to alleviate underlying anxiety.
2. Care for the thermodilution catheter is the same as that outlined for PA catheterization.
3. Make sure stopcocks are well secured and turned in the precise direction to avoid showering the patient with injectate.
4. Maintain the sterility of the injectate by using injectate-filled syringes not more than 4 hours old.
5. Account for injectate volume in the intake and output record.
6. Monitor the patient's fluid status, daily weights, edema, gallop rhythm, intake and output and serum sodium values. Patients with a compromised myocardium are at risk of fluid overload from frequent thermodilution CO determinations.
7. Methods of troubleshooting problems in thermodilution measurements are outlined in Table 7–3.

CENTRAL VENOUS PRESSURE (CVP) MONITORING

Definition

Central venous pressure monitoring is defined as measurement of the pressure exerted by blood against the walls of the right atrium or great veins of the thorax or both.

Rationale

Central venous pressure is determined by vascular tone, blood volume and the ability of the right heart to receive and

Table 7–3. TROUBLESHOOTING PROBLEMS OF THERMODILUTION MEASUREMENTS

PROBLEM	POSSIBLE CAUSE
1. Large variability of CO reading	1. a. Injectate rate is too low. Ten ml must be delivered within 4 seconds. b. Injectate is rewarmed by handling syringe barrel. c. Intermittent positive pressure ventilation or PEEP >15 cm H_2O causes variation in PA temperature. d. Excessive movement of the patient's extremities causes return of cooled blood, thus lowering the PA temperature. e. Temperature probe of bath is not accurate. f. Baseline PA temperature may be unstable, with fluctuations >0.6° C (may be observed with strip-chart recording). g. Thermistor bead may be wedged against the PA wall.
2. Unusually high reading	2. The volume of injectate is less than computer calibration.
3. Unusually low reading	3. The volume of injectate is more than computer calibration.
4. No digital display	4. a. Computer battery is depleted. b. Thermodilution catheter may be nonfunctioning (fractured thermistor wires).

pump blood. A change in any one of these determinants may cause the CVP change also.

Procedure

With sterile technique, a catheter is introduced into the right atrium or thoracic venae cavae via the subclavian, jugular, innominate, saphenous or antecubital vein by percutaneous puncture or cutdown. The indwelling catheter is then connected to one of the following:

1. A pressurized transducer system set up for continuous pressure monitoring (RA port on balloon-tip, flow-directed thermodilution catheter).
2. A water manometer with a three-way stopcock for intermittent pressure monitoring.

If a water manometer is to be used, the level of the right atrium must be determined as a zero point to obtain a correct measurement. With the patient in supine position, this is located at the fourth interspace and the midaxillary line. Mark this spot clearly on the patient with tape or felt-tip pen. All readings should be taken at this level.

To obtain a reading via the water manometer:

1. Check the catheter for patency by allowing the intravenous fluid to run rapidly for a brief period (Fig. 7–6A).
2. Turn the manometer stopcock off to the patient and open to the intravenous (IV) infusion and the manometer. Run the fluid level in the column up to around the 25-cm level (Fig. 7–6B).
3. Turn the stopcock off to the IV infusion and open to the manometer and the patient, allowing the solution to flow from the manometer into the CVP line (Fig. 7–6C). Initially, there is a smooth, rapid drop in the fluid level, followed by an overall stop in downward movement. However, the fluid level should continue to fluctuate a few centimeters with the patient's respiration. The reading is then taken when the fluid column in the manometer reaches its highest point in fluctuation. Normal values are 4 to 10 cm of water.
4. Turn the stopcock off to the manometer and open to the patient and the IV infusion. Adjust the IV rate (Fig. 7–6A).

Indications

This may be performed in any condition in which there is a need to assess right heart hemodynamics, volume status or

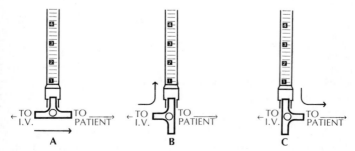

Figure 7–6. CVP measurement and stopcock directions of manometer. *A,* Stopcock position during IV infusion. *B,* Stopcock position during filling of the manometer. *C,* Stopcock position during taking of a reading.

vascular tone. See Table 7–4 for listed indications as well as how they may be expected to affect the CVP reading. A CVP line may also be used for blood drawing (routine laboratory work as well as determination of venous oxygen saturation), administration of medications that are caustic to peripheral veins and infusion of fluids.

Complications

1. Pneumothorax
2. Vein trauma
3. Phlebitis
4. Displacement or improper positioning of catheter
5. Air emboli
6. Pulmonary emboli
7. Fluid overload
8. Arrhythmia
9. Infection
10. Electromicro shock

Nursing Management

Preprocedure

    a. Explain the procedure and its purpose to the patient.
    b. Position the patient in a supine or Trendelenburg (if using central approach) position.
    c. Prep the skin at the future insertion site per unit protocol.
    d. Assemble the equipment and preflush tubings.

Table 7–4. INDICATIONS FOR CVP AND HOW THEY MAY AFFECT THE READINGS

	↑ CVP (>10 cm H_2O)	↓ CVP (<4 cm H_2O)
Right heart hemodynamics	Right heart failure (including chronic CHF, LVF)* Constrictive pericarditis Cardiac tamponade Valvular stenosis Pulmonary hypertension	Early LVF
Blood volume	↑ Circulating volume	↓ Circulating volume
Vascular tone	Vasoconstriction Hypertension	Vasodilation/peripheral pooling Septic shock

*CHF, congestive heart failure; LVF, left ventricular failure.

Postprocedure

Check for Proper Positioning of the Catheter and Possible Pneumothorax

   i. Obtain a chest X-ray immediately after insertion.
   ii. Auscultate all lung fields for the presence of breath sounds, rales or rhonchi.
   iii. Watch for arrhythmias.

Keep the Line Patent

   i. Check the IV rate frequently to avoid fluid overload or obstruction.
   ii. If obstruction to flow occurs, check for kinks in the catheter. Always aspirate before irrigating. Never irrigate against resistance to flow.
   iii. Secure and tape all connections.

Maintain Accurate Readings

   i. Patient should always be supine for readings. If patient is unable to assume the supine position, record the lowest position that he or she can assume and take all readings with the head of the bed at that elevation (e.g., 30 degrees).
   ii. All readings should be taken from the same zero point. Make sure it is clearly marked.
   iii. If the patient is on a ventilator, it is preferable that he or she be taken off briefly to obtain an accurate CVP reading. Record whether the patient is on or off the ventilator at the time of reading so that all subsequent readings may be done the same way.
   iv. The column of water in the manometer should fluctuate with the patient's respirations. If fluctuation is absent, check the catheter for kinks and the manometer for fluid overflow.

Prevent Infection

   i. Good dressing care with strict aseptic technique is mandatory. Wear sterile gloves. Use povidone-iodine (Betadine) or other antiseptic at the puncture site; cleanse it with alcohol and apply povidone-iodine (Betadine) or other antibacterial ointment. Inspect the puncture site for redness, edema and drainage. Change the dressing daily.

   ii. Change all tubing, including the manometer and IV solution every 24 hours.

  iii. If the fluid level in the manometer overflows, change the manometer.

Monitor the Patient. Do this as necessary, observing for significant changes. Watch for a trend in the values obtained rather than for a change in a single reading.

INTRA-ARTERIAL MONITORING (Arterial Line)

Definition

Intra-arterial monitoring is defined as the continuous detection of arterial blood pressure via an indwelling catheter.

Rationale

In patients with low cardiac output and excessive peripheral vasoconstriction or rapid changes, the Korotkoff's sound of the conventional cuff blood pressure (BP) measurement cannot be heard owing to low stroke volume. Therefore, accurate blood pressure measurement is not obtainable except by direct intra-arterial detection.

General Procedure

A short indwelling catheter is introduced into an artery (radial, brachial, axillary, femoral or even dorsalis pedis) through a needle insertion using sterile technique. The catheter is then connected to a transducer and a monitor for pressure takings. The transducer converts the arterial pressure to electrical wave forms (Fig. 7–7), which are displayed on the monitor oscilloscope. The systolic, diastolic and mean

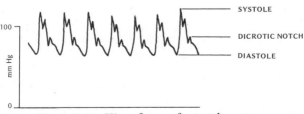

Figure 7–7. Wave forms of arterial pressure.

pressures can also be obtained from the digital display. The entire monitoring system is maintained patent by continuous infusion of heparinized IV solution under pressure.

Indications

Intra-arterial monitoring is needed whenever frequent blood pressure measurement becomes necessary or accurate blood pressure measurement is difficult to obtain, such as during cardiac surgery or in patients with shock or in those receiving vasodilators or vasopressors. It may also be utilized for patients who need frequent blood samples for arterial blood gas evaluation.

Complications

Clot Formation.   This may occur at the catheter tip or on the inner surface of the catheter.

Diminished or Absent Pulse Distal to the Insertion Site. This is caused by occlusion of the artery that supplies the distal portion of the extremity.

Hemorrhage.   This is usually caused by loose connections of the monitoring system. It may bleed back into the tubing, dome and transducer.

Hematoma at the Insertion Site.   This may occur after removal of the catheter.

Infection.   This may be localized or systemic (sepsis). It is caused by inadequate, aseptic technique used during the insertion or monitoring period. Prolonged catheterization may also predispose to infection.

Nursing Management

Preprocedure

   a. Explain the purpose and procedure of arterial cathet-
      erization to the patient, including the fact that it will
      alleviate the need for further arterial punctures.
   b. Prepare the skin at and around the puncture site by
      following individual hospital protocol.
   c. If the radial artery is chosen for catheter insertion,
      the blood flow of the hand should be evaluated by
      performing an Allen's test: Occlude both radial and

ulnar arteries at the wrist. Have the patient make a tight fist. Release the pressure over the ulnar artery. Have the patient open the hand. If the fingers become pink rapidly, it indicates adequate ulnar circulation.

Postprocedure

Monitor and Record Blood Pressure Hourly or as Indicated. This is accomplished by reading the digital display as well as by observing the wave forms. For accurate reading, the transducer should be kept at the same level as the insertion site. The monitoring system should be adequately connected and securely taped. The system should be free of clots and air bubbles. Both may lead to damped tracing. The equipment should be properly calibrated every 4 hours or as required by institution policy.

Maintain Patency of the Catheter. By using the combination of a pressure bag (300 mm Hg) and a continuous flushing device, the catheter is infused with heparinized IV fluid, 2 to 5 ml per hour. After each drawing of a blood sample, the catheter should be flushed. If the wave form is damped and thrombus is suspected, the line should be aspirated before flushing for fear of embolism.

Monitor Circulation Distal to the Insertion Site. This is accomplished by frequent detection of pulse, color, temperature and sensation at the distal portion of the extremity. Any change may indicate impairment of circulation and impending arterial occlusion.

Prevent and Correct Damped Tracing. This may be done by keeping the catheter free from clots, repositioning the catheter, maintaining alignment of the extremity and avoiding tight dressing above the insertion site.

Prevent Hemorrhage. Hemorrhage can be avoided by taping all connections securely. The catheterized extremity should be kept uncovered for easy observation of the insertion site and the connecting tubings. A built-in alarm is helpful for detecting breaks in the system. The catheter should be sutured in place to prevent accidental advancement or withdrawal.

Prevent Infection. This can be done by using strict aseptic technique whenever the tubing, IV fluid or dressing needs to be changed. Ordinarily, they are changed daily. If the dome or transducer becomes contaminated, it should also be replaced. During each dressing change, the insertion site should be inspected carefully, and antibacterial ointment should be applied. Catheterization should be limited to less than 96 hours.

Obtain Arterial Blood Sample. This blood sample can be obtained by aspirating blood from the stopcock nearest to the insertion site. Caution should be used not to contaminate or dislodge the line. The sample is obtained after discarding the initial few ml (up to 5 ml) of blood, which are mixed with IV fluid. The entire line, including the sample port, should then be flushed thoroughly.

Prevent Hematoma. Hematoma may be avoided by maintaining firm pressure for 10 minutes and applying a pressure dressing to the insertion site after the catheter is removed.

SUGGESTED READINGS

Daily, E. K., and Schroeder, J. S.: *Techniques in Bedside Hemodynamic Monitoring*, 2nd ed. St. Louis, C. V. Mosby, 1981.

Dizon, C., Gerazi, W., Barash, P., and Crittenden, J.: Hand held thermo-dilution cardiac output injector. *Crit. Care Med.* 5:210, 1977.

Edwards Laboratories: *Swan-Ganz Monitoring Systems*. Santa Ana, Edwards Laboratory, 1977.

Fiker, E.: Measuring central venous pressure. *Nursing '79*, 9:74, 1979.

Forrester, J. S., et al.: Hemodynamic therapy of myocardial infarction. *N. Engl. J. Med.*, 295:1356, 1976.

Haughey, B.: CVP lines: monitoring and maintaining. *AJN*, 78:635, 1978.

Lamb, J.: Intra-arterial monitoring. *Nursing '77*, 7:65, 1977.

Murray, J., and Smallwood, J.: Monitoring. *Nursing '77*, 7:42, 1977.

Pugh, D. A.: Thermodilution cardiac output: What, how and why. *Crit. Care Q.* 2:21, 1979.

8

CARDIAC CATHETERIZATION AND ANGIOGRAPHY

DEFINITION

Cardiac Catheterization

Cardiac catheterization involves the insertion of a radiopaque catheter via a peripheral artery or vein into the heart for determining hemodynamic function and for performing angiography. The patient is under local anesthesia for this procedure.

Cardiac Angiography

Cardiac angiography is the radiographical visualization of the heart, coronary arteries and great vessels achieved by injecting radiopaque contrast media through a cardiac catheter at various selected sites. Serial X-ray pictures (angiograms) are usually taken during the procedure for permanent reference.

TYPES

Right Cardiac Catheterization

The catheter is inserted through the antecubital or femoral vein. Under fluoroscopic guidance, the catheter is advanced slowly to the right atrium and right ventricle and finally is wedged in a small branch of the pulmonary artery. Right cardiac catheterization is usually performed in the catheterization laboratory. However, it may also be carried out at the bedside in the Critical Care Unit by using a thermistor-tipped balloon flotation catheter (see Chapter 7).

Left Cardiac Catheterization

Arterial Approach. The catheter is introduced via an artery (femoral or brachial). It is advanced, in a retrograde fashion, to the aorta and left ventricle.

Transseptal Approach. Via right cardiac catheterization approach, the atrial septum is punctured, and left cardiac catheterization is then accomplished. This approach is used when a diseased mitral valve is suspected.

Right Cardiac Angiography

The radiopaque contrast medium is injected at the following sites.

Superior or Inferior Vena Cava. This site is used for detecting the thickness of the walls of the atria, Ebstein's malformation of the tricuspid valve, or tricuspid atresia.

Right Ventricle (Right Ventriculography). The right ventricle is injected for determining pulmonic stenosis and tetralogy of Fallot.

Main Pulmonary Artery. This site is used for detecting pulmonary thromboemboli and congenital pulmonary anomalies.

Left Cardiac Angiography (Left Ventriculography)

The contrast medium is injected in the left ventricle to examine the mitral valve, the outflow tract of the ventricle, wall motion and thickness, mural thrombi, left ventricular end-diastolic volume and ejection fraction.

Ascending Aortography

The contrast medium is injected in the aorta to determine the severity of aortic valve regurgitation and the size and location of the aortic aneurysm.

Coronary Arteriography

The medium is injected directly into each coronary artery to visualize atherosclerotic lesions, coronary arteriovenous fistulas, congenital abnormalities and collateral vessels.

INDICATIONS

Cardiac catheterization and angiography are often used in patients with congenital heart disease, acquired valvular disease, angina, idiopathic hypertrophic subaortic stenosis, pulmonary hypertension, recurrent symptoms following cardiac surgery, congestive heart failure and hypotension after acute myocardial infarction (MI) (continuous hemodynamic monitoring) to establish diagnosis and quantitate any anatomic or hemodynamic defect. Other indications include endocardial biopsy, intracardiac electrocardiogram (ECG) or phonogram, and injection of streptokinase into the coronary artery following acute myocardial infarction.

INFORMATION PROVIDED BY CARDIAC CATHETERIZATION AND ANGIOGRAPHY

1. Anatomy of the cardiac chambers, valves, great vessels and coronary arteries.
2. Spatial relationship of atria, ventricles and the great vessels.
3. Ventricular wall thickness and motions.
4. Intracardiac and intravascular pressures and pressure gradients across the valves.
5. Cardiac output.
6. Myocardial function.
7. Oxygen saturation in different chambers.
8. Intracardiac shunts.
9. Coronary blood flow.
10. Pulmonary system and vascular resistance.

CONTRAINDICATIONS

1. Cardiac catheterization is not indicated if the same diagnostic information can be obtained by using other noninvasive, less expensive and risky procedures.
2. It is not used if the information obtained will not improve the management of the patient.
3. It should not be carried out in patients with ventricular irritability, hypertension, elevated temperature, anemia, digitalis toxicity and electrolyte imbalance.

COMPLICATIONS

Perforation of the Heart and Great Vessels

Perforation may be associated with excessive catheter manipulation. It may lead to cardiac tamponade.

Hemorrhage or Hematoma

These may occur retroperitoneally or at the insertion site.

Arrhythmias

Atrial and ventricular tachycardia or fibrillation may result from irritation of the heart. Severe bradycardia and heart block may result from parasympathetic response to pain or anxiety.

Hypotension

Hypotension is due to parasympathetic response. It may lead to severe arrhythmia and shock.

Vascular Thrombosis

Thrombosis occurs especially at the site of arteriotomy. It may progress to cerebral embolism or vascular occlusion.

Myocardial Infarction

Myocardial infarction is usually associated with left ventriculography or coronary arteriography.

Reaction to the Contrast Media

Reaction to contrast media ranges from urticaria to convulsive seizures.

Pyrogenic Reaction

This type of reaction results from contamination with a foreign substance. It is characterized by shaking, chills and increase of body temperature.

Death

The primary risk is related to the severity of the cardiac disease.

NURSING MANAGEMENT

Preprocedure

1. The procedure should be explained to the patient. If necessary, the patient is taken to the laboratory and introduced to the personnel and surroundings. The pa-

tient should also be forewarned about the sound made by the X-ray apparatus during the procedure.

2. An informed consent should be obtained.
3. The patient is told that other than the injection of local anesthetics, the procedure is not painful. However, the patient may experience some discomfort owing to the length of the procedure. He or she may also have a warm-to-hot sensation whenever the contrast medium is injected.
4. The patient may have nothing by mouth for 4 to 8 hours before the procedure or have a light liquid breakfast if the procedure is scheduled in the afternoon.
5. Sedatives are given as prescribed.
6. A prophylactic antibiotic agent may be given.
7. Diphenhydramine (Benadryl), 25 to 50 mg, may be given to prevent a hypersensitivity reaction.
8. Atropine, 0.4 mg, may be administered to prevent severe bradycardia.
9. The skin of the insertion site should be shaved and prepared.

Postprocedure

1. Take vital signs every 15 minutes initially and then less frequently, as specified by the institution policy.
2. Check the pressure dressing and watch for excessive bleeding at the puncture site.
3. Check pulse, color, warmth and feelings of the extremity distal to the insertion site.
4. Monitor cardiac rhythm and treat arrhythmias as needed.
5. Strict bed rest should be maintained for at least 6 hours with a sandbag applied to the groin if the femoral approach has been used.
6. Give analgesics as needed.
7. Encourage fluid intake (2 to 3 liters/6 to 8 hours) for adequate elimination of the contrast media.
8. Help the patient to understand the findings of the test.

SUGGESTED READINGS

Bogart, D. B., and Pugh, D. M.: Cardiac catheterization complications: diagnosis and management. *Journal of Cardiovascular and Pulmonary Technique*, 5:25, 1977.

Braunwald, E.: *Heart Disease.* Philadelphia, W. B. Saunders, 1980.
Gilbert, C. J., and Akhtar, M.: Right heart catheterization for intracardiac electrophysiologic studies: implication for the primary care nurse. *Heart and Lung,* 9:85, 1980.
Karimian, H. O., et al.: The clinical importance of coronary arteriography after myocardial infarction. *Heart and Lung,* 8:87, 1979.
Schoonmaker, F. W., and Vijay, M. K.: Why coronary angiography? *Journal of Cardiovascular and Pulmonary Techniques,* 5:15, 1977.
Strong, A. B.: Caring for cardiac catheterization patients. *Nursing '77,* 60:4, 1977.

9

ECHOCARDIOGRAPHY

DEFINITION

Echocardiography is a noninvasive method of recording cardiac structure and motion via the echo (reflection) of pulsed ultrasound.

MODES

1. With A (amplitude) mode, echoes are indicated by spikes; the more intense the echo, the greater the amplitude of the spike.
2. In B (brightness) mode, echoes are indicated by dots; the more intense the echo, the brighter the dot.
3. With M (motion) mode, echoes are displayed in a time-motion relationship by sweeping the B mode with respect to time.
4. In cross-sectional mode (real-time or two-dimensional sector scan), a computer or microprocessor controls the firing and direction of a very rapid ultrasonic beam, resulting in depiction of cardiac shape and lateral motion, which is recorded on videotape or movie film.
5. With Doppler mode, continuous-wave ultrasound energy is combined with pulse ultrasound, resulting not only in imaging of the heart but also in assessment of directional blood flow.

MECHANISM

An echo is produced when ultrasonic waves, sent and received by a transducer (microphone), bounce off tissues of different densities and thus create an image via an oscilloscope graph. The bursts of ultrasound are directed at the part of the heart to be studied, and the echocardiogram records the structure and motion of the area in relation to its distance from the anterior chest wall. An electrocardiogram (ECG) is recorded simultaneously on the graph. See Figure 9–1.

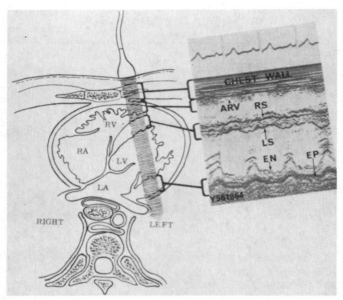

Figure 9–1. Echocardiogram obtained from an anteroposterior view of the heart. (From Braunwald, E. (ed.): *Heart Disease.* Philadelphia, W. B. Saunders, 1980. Modified from Popp, R. L., et al.: Estimation of right and left ventricular size by ultrasound. A study of the echoes from the interventricular septum. *Am. J. Cardiol.*, 24:523, 1969.)

INDICATIONS

Echocardiography is used for the diagnosis or assessment of the following:

Cardiomyopathies	Abnormalities of the great vessels
Cardiac tumors	Left ventricular function
Pericardial effusion	Coronary artery disease
Valvular heart disease	Myocardial ischemia
Cardiac shunts	Ventricular aneurysms

NURSING MANAGEMENT

1. Reassure the patient that the procedure is noninvasive, painless and without complication.
2. Explain the procedure and the need for it to the patient.
3. Alert the patient to the time the procedure is scheduled.

SUGGESTED READINGS

Braunwald, E.: *Heart Disease*. Philadelphia, W. B. Saunders, 1980.

Naggar, C. Z.: Ultrasound in medical diagnosis. Part I: Applications in cardiology. *Heart and Lung*, 5:6, 1976.

Parisi, A. F., et al.: Noninvasive cardiac diagnosis. *N. Engl. J. Med.*, 296:316, 368, 427, 1977.

Rasmussen, S., and Corya, B.: The diagnostic attributes of echocardiography in the patient with chest pain or pulmonary edema. *Heart and Lung*, 6:4, 1977.

DEFINITION

Myocardial scintigraphy is a method of directly assessing myocardial perfusion via radionuclide imaging.

MODES

1. In "cold spot" scanning, the radioactive agent, most commonly thallium 201 (Tl), concentrates in normal myocardial cells. A normal image shows uniform distribution of Tl throughout the left ventricle. This test is done at rest or under stress (exercise).
   a. An infarcted myocardium shows a lack of Tl uptake at rest as well as under stress.
   b. An ischemic myocardium may show Tl uptake at rest but a decrease in or absence of Tl uptake under stress.
2. In "hot spot" scanning, the radioactive agent, most commonly technetium 99m stannous pyrophosphate (^{99m}Tc-PYP), concentrates in recently infarcted myocardial cells. A normal image shows no significant uptake of ^{99m}Tc-PYP in the region of the heart.

MECHANISM

When specific radiopharmaceuticals are given (intravenously), they emit photons that are externally detectable, resulting in a radionuclide image.
1. In "cold spot" scanning, Tl concentrates in normal myocardial cells via coronary blood flow and diffusion and exchange with potassium (Na-K-ATPase system).
2. In "hot spot" scanning, the exact mechanism for concentration of ^{99m}Tc-PYP in infarcted myocardial cells is controversial. One theory suggests that ^{99m}Tc-PYP accumulates in a damaged myocardium in association with the presence of calcium deposits.

Table 10–1. INDICATIONS FOR MYOCARDIAL SCINTIGRAPHY

"COLD SPOT" SCANNING	"HOT SPOT" SCANNING
1. As an adjunct to exercise ECG when results are equivocal. 2. Evaluation of atypical chest pain. 3. Evaluation of suspected coronary artery disease in patient with abnormal resting ECG. 4. As an adjunct to coronary angiography when there is question about the significance of a stenotic lesion. 5. Confirmation of coronary artery patency after coronary artery bypass graft surgery or percutaneous transluminal coronary artery dilation.	1. As an adjunct to ECG and enzyme analysis in diagnosis of acute MI when results are otherwise equivocal or after cardiac surgery. 2. Aids in diagnosis of acute MI in patient with left bundle branch block (LBBB). 3. Demonstration of small transmural infarcts. 4. Demonstration of extension of MI or new MI in patient with recent infarct. 5. Demonstration of myocardial contusion.

INDICATIONS

See Table 10–1 for specific uses of myocardial scintigraphy.
1. "Cold spot" scanning is used for the detection and evaluation of myocardial cell ischemia and necrosis.
2. "Hot spot" scanning aids in the detection, localization and quantification of acute myocardial infarction.

NURSING MANAGEMENT

The patient should be managed as for echocardiography.

SUGGESTED READINGS

Alpert, J. S., and Rippe, J. M.: *Manual of Cardiovascular Diagnosis and Therapy.* Boston, Little, Brown and Co., 1980.
Braunwald, E.: *Heart Disease.* Philadelphia, W. B. Saunders, 1980.
Callen, I. R. (ed.): Noninvasive cardiac diagnosis I. *Med. Clin. North Am.,* 64:1, 1980.
Callen, I. R. (ed.): Noninvasive cardiac diagnosis II. *Med. Clin. North Am.,* 64:2, 1980.
Parisi, A. F., et al.: Noninvasive cardiac diagnosis. *N. Engl. J. Med.,* 296:316, 368, 427, 1977.

III

CARDIAC DISORDERS

11

CARDIOVASCULAR DISORDERS

_____ **Coronary Atherosclerosis** _____

DEFINITION

Atherosclerosis is narrowing of the arteries caused by proliferation of cells and accumulaton of lipids in large and middle-sized arteries. The aorta, femoral, cerebral and coronary arteries are affected most often.

PREVALENCE

Atherosclerosis is the process underlying most heart disease and is the leading cause of death in the United States. Although statistics show a decline in deaths from coronary artery disease, still over one-half million Americans die from this cause each year.

PATHOGENESIS

The true pathogenesis of atherosclerosis is unknown, although family tendencies and certain risk factors are highly associated with its occurrence. The atherosclerotic process involves the formation of three lesions. (See Fig. 11–1.)

1. The *fatty streak* is a yellow, smooth lesion that protrudes into the intima and is present in many young people and infants.
2. The raised *fibrous plaque* is a yellowish, gray lump that protrudes into the intima from the medial layer and sometimes obstructs blood flow. It results from proliferation of smooth muscle and collagen and lipid accumulation and is the lesion of coronary artery disease.
3. The *complicated lesion* results when there has been hemorrhage into a fibrous plaque and the clot calcifies. It is most often associated with myocardial infarction.

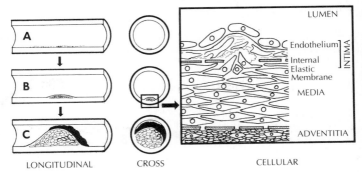

Figure 11–1. Lesions of the atherosclerotic process. *A*, Fatty streak. *B*, Fibrous plaque. *C*, Complicated lesion.

RISK FACTORS

Several risk factors are thought to accelerate the atherosclerotic process and the development of CAD. Risk factors are classified as modifiable and unmodifiable, for purposes of identifying the factors that the patient can control or modify.

Modifiable Risk Factors

The three major modifiable risk factors associated with coronary artery disease are *cigarette smoking, hypertension,* and *elevated serum cholesterol levels*. Other modifiable risk factors are diabetes, thyroid dysfunction, obesity, sedentary lifestyle, stress, behavior predisposing to coronary artery disease, caffeine, and the use of oral contraceptives.

Unmodifiable Risk Factors

Age.   Susceptibility to atherosclerosis increases with age. Significant disease before age 40 is unusual.

Gender.   Women are relatively immune to atherosclerosis before menopause.

Family Tendency.   A family history of coronary artery disease is one of the strongest risk factors, especially when the disease has occurred in siblings or parents under 50 years of age.

MANIFESTATIONS

The three most common manifestations of coronary artery atherosclerosis are angina, myocardial infarction and sudden cardiac death.

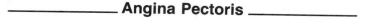

Angina Pectoris

GENERAL CONSIDERATIONS

Definition

Angina pectoris is a symptom of transient myocardial ischemia perceived by the patient as chest pain or discomfort.

Classification

Stable (Chronic) Angina.   This is an effort-induced discomfort that has not changed in duration, intensity or frequency for at least 2 months. It can be mild or debilitating.

Unstable (Acute) Angina.   This differs from stable angina in that it is a *changing* pattern of discomfort. The following terms are used to describe various forms of unstable angina:
Crescendo Angina.   This is an effort-induced pain that occurs with increasing frequency and with decreasing provocation.
Progressive Angina.   This is a newly acquired angina that rapidly progresses in severity.
Pre-infarction Angina.   This is a term for unstable angina that progresses to myocardial infarction.
Angina Decubitus.   The patient experiences this pain at rest upon assuming a recumbent position.
Nocturnal Angina.   The onset of this pain is associated with rapid eye movement (REM) during sleep.

Prinzmetal's (Variant) Angina.   This is a severe, non–effort-induced pain that occurs at rest without provocation and may be of greater duration than other types of angina. It is often cyclical in fashion and may occur at the same time each day. It differs from other forms of angina in that it is more often seen in women under 50 years of age and is attributed to spasms of a large coronary artery.

ETIOLOGY

Precipitating Factors

Angina pectoris is primarily a manifestation of coronary atherosclerosis, although, in rare instances, it may occur without significant atherosclerotic changes. See Figure 11–2 for precipitating factors.

Cause

The underlying cause for angina pectoris is a disequilibrium between myocardial oxygen demands and oxygen supply. The resulting myocardial ischemia is transient and, unlike myocardial infarction, does not lead to tissue necrosis.

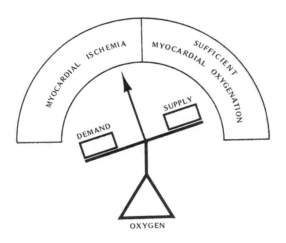

FACTORS THAT INCREASE OXYGEN DEMAND	FACTORS THAT DECREASE OXYGEN SUPPLY
Hypertension	Atherosclerosis
Stress	Coronary arteritis/trauma
Temperature extremes	Hypotension (shock)
Exercise	Severe tachycardia/bradycardia
Smoking	Anemia
Aortic stenosis	Aortic stenosis/insufficiency
Thyrotoxicosis	Hypoxemia
Pheochromocytosis	Polycythemia vera
Heavy meals	Smoking

Figure 11–2. Precipitating factors of angina and oxygen demand-supply relationships.

Myocardial Oxygen Demands.　Oxygen requirements of the heart are greater than those of most other body tissues and are directly related to the workload of the heart. This workload is, in turn, determined by preload, afterload, heart rate and myocardial contractility. An increase in any one of these factors can greatly augment myocardial oxygen demands.

Myocardial Oxygen Supply.　Diseased arteries cannot respond to increased myocardial oxygen demands and hypoxia with dilation and increased perfusion (autoregulation). An atherosclerotic lesion producing an obstruction of 75 to 80 per cent in at least one coronary artery must exist before blood flow is impeded to the point of symptomatic myocardial ischemia. Diminished myocardial perfusion may also result from sympathetic reflex vasoconstriction, increased blood viscosity and an excessive fall in blood pressure.

PATHOPHYSIOLOGY

Ischemia

Transient myocardial ischemia will result in significant but reversible cellular changes. Inadequate oxygen supply forces the myocardium to shift from aerobic metabolism to a less efficient anaerobic metabolism. The resultant decrease in energy substrate, lactic acid accumulation and possible reduction in calcium release from the endoplasmic reticulum may rapidly impair myocardial function and alter hemodynamics. The end result may be a transient decrease in stroke volume and cardiac output, with increasing left ventricular end-diastolic volume. This increase in preload can add to myocardial oxygen demands, further taxing the ischemic heart.

Pain

Pain associated with angina pectoris is thought to be due to anoxia and to the accumulation of metabolites, particularly potent vasodilators like kinins, histamines, and prostaglandins. Myocardial ischemia is detected by small sensory nerves that are associated with the autonomic nerves and enter the spinal cord at the C4 and T8 segments. Like all visceral pain, it is poorly localized and is usually referred to the C8 to T4 dermatomes. The thumb is innervated by C5 and C6 der-

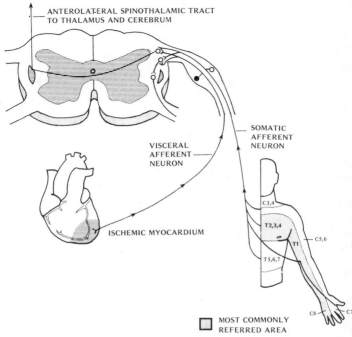

ANTEROLATERAL SPINOTHALAMIC TRACT
TO THALAMUS AND CEREBRUM

SOMATIC
AFFERENT
NEURON

VISCERAL
AFFERENT
NEURON

ISCHEMIC MYOCARDIUM

C3,4

T2,3,4

C5,6

T1

T5,6,7

C8

C7

MOST COMMONLY
REFERRED AREA

Figure 11–3. Mechanisms of referred cardiac pain in the derma-tomes.

matomes and is rarely involved in anginal pain. (See Fig. 11–3).

PATIENT ASSESSMENT

History-Taking

The diagnosis of angina is based on the patient's descriptions of anginal episodes.

Data Regarding Previous Episodes

Frequency. A history should be obtained regarding the frequency of anginal attacks and recent tendencies toward increase in frequency, duration or intensity. An increase in anginal attacks can be indicated by a rise in the number of nitroglycerin tablets the patient requires weekly at the present time compared with 6 months ago.

Initial Attack. Data should include when the initial attack occurred and when angina was first medically documented.

Data Regarding Current Episode

Duration. Duration of the pain is an important differentiating symptom. Pain described as fleeting is usually muscular in origin. Anginal pain is usually 3 to 10 minutes in duration.

Location. The location of anginal pain is usually substernal or left precordial and often radiates down the left arm. It is sometimes described as being in the jaw or fingertips. It is usually not felt in the thumb.

Quality. The quality of anginal pain is varied. It may be described as gripping, aching, pressing or burning and is rarely stabbing. It may be felt only as a tingling in the fingers. Although the pain is unique to each patient, they usually learn to differentiate their cardiac pain. The patient may deny pain but admit to chest discomfort, belching, indigestion, pressure, tightness or tingling.

Intensity. Anginal pain is usually described as 5 or less on a rating scale of 1 to 10.

Precipitating Factors. Angina is classically related to exertion, with the exception of Printzmetal's angina. The patient should be questioned as to what events occurred prior to the anginal attack.

Alleviating Factors. The patient should be asked what alleviated the pain, whether it was rest, antacids or nitroglycerin. It is important to ascertain how many nitroglycerin tablets were needed to terminate the attack.

Lifestyle

A history regarding lifestyle shold include identification of risk factors and impact on the patient's activities of daily living. The impact of angina on the patient's activites should be assessed by discussion focusing on limitations of self-care and of recreational activities and amount of dependence on others for care. Discrepancies between lifestyle desired and lifestyle lived should be identified.

Physical Examination

The patient's clinical appearance should be noted, both during anginal episodes and during nonsymptomatic states. The following symptoms may be manifested during an anginal attack: dyspnea, diaphoresis, cold and clammy skin, increased heart rate, pulsus alternans, transiently abnormal point of maximal impulse (PMI), an S_4 gallop, a rare transient systolic murmur and, most frequently, anxiety.

Diagnostic Tests

Diagnostic tests include those that differentiate angina from myocardial infarction and those that document coronary artery disease.

Cardiac Enzymes. These are assessed to rule out myocardial infarction.

Complete Blood Count (CBC). This is done to rule out anemia-induced angina.

Electrocardiogram. An electrocardiogram (ECG) may document transient ischemic changes during anginal episodes. Ischemia is evidenced by ST depression or T-wave inversion (Fig. 11–4). Prinzmetal's angina appears as marked ST segment elevation during pain (see Fig. 11–5).

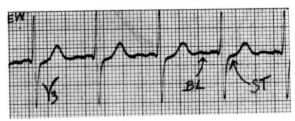

Initial tracing

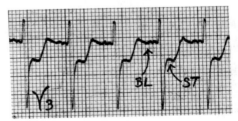

Tracing during
anginal attack

Figure 11–4. ECG changes of angina. *A,* Initial tracing. *B,* Tracing during anginal attack. (From Phillips, R. E., and Feeney, M. K.: *The Cardiac Rhythms,* 2nd ed. Philadelphia, W. B. Saunders, 1980.)

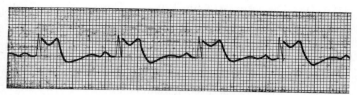

DURING CHEST PAIN

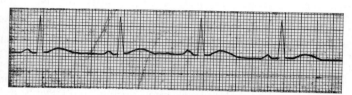

AFTER PAIN IS RELIEVED

Figure 11–5. ECG changes of prinzmetal angina.

Echocardiogram. An echocardiogram is performed to rule out aortic valvular disease and idiopathic hypertrophic subaortic stenosis.

Exercise Testing. This testing is used to reproduce an episode or to induce ST changes to provide electrocardiographic evidence of myocardial ischemia.

Angiography. This procedure is indicated to document coronary artery disease and to facilitate selection of treatment.

COMPLICATIONS

Complications of Angina Pectoris

Psychological Stress. Fear and worry associated with chest pain increase with repeated attacks of angina. Both pain and psychological stress limit the patient's activity level or desire to participate and may even incapacitate some patients.

Myocardial Infarction. Approximately one in every three patients with angina pectoris will eventually develop myocardial infarction.

Arrhythmia. Ventricular irritability secondary to myocardial ischemia can lead to sudden death.

Treatment-Induced Complications

Induced by Nitrates
Headache.   Headache may be mild or severe; it is caused by cerebral vasodilation.
Postural Hypotension.   This is caused by peripheral vasodilation. The patient may become syncopal.
Reflex Tachycardia.   This disorder often results as a response to hypotension.

Induced by Beta-Blocker
Congestive heart failure is caused by the negative inotropic effect of the beta-blockers, e.g., propranolol. Other complications that can result from beta blockade include bradycardia, postural hypotension and depression.

Induced by Calcium Channel Blocker
Congestive heart failure, edema, headache and flushing can result from use of drugs that act as calcium channel blockers.

MEDICAL AND NURSING MANAGEMENT

Rest
Rest of both the body and the mind decreases oxygen demands of the heart. Pain is often relieved by immediate cessation of the physical activity that precipitated the attack. Sedation for emotional stress may also be indicated. Activities that are known to precipitate attacks should be avoided if possible.

Change of Position
Change from a supine to a sitting or standing position will often alleviate anginal pain by decreasing central blood volume and thus reducing the heart's demand for oxygen.

Nitrates
Nitrates decrease myocardial oxygen demands by causing a reduction in preload and afterload. They also may increase oxygen supply to the myocardium by dilation of the coronary arteries and their collateral circulation. On an emergency basis, a sublingual nitroglycerin tablet (0.15 to 0.6 mg) usually relieves anginal pain within 1 to 2 minutes, having a duration of 30 minutes. Sublingual nitroglycerin is also used prophy-

lactically, before the patient engages in activities that are known to precipitate anginal attacks. Longer acting prophylactic nitrate therapy is available in pill form, such as isosorbide dinitrate (Isordil) (2.5 to 30 mg qid), or in a 2 per cent ointment form, such as Nitropaste (spread in ½- to 5-inch area, q 4 to 6 hours). Both demonstrate an antianginal effect of approximately 6 hours.

Beta-Blockers

Beta-blockers such as propranolol (Inderal), 10 to 20 mg tid or qid (other beta blockers are discussed in Chapter 17), decrease oxygen consumption of the myocardium by decreasing heart rate, blood pressure and myocardial contractility. The actions of nitrates and beta-blockers complement each other.

Calcium Channel Blockers

Blockers such as verapamil (5 to 10 mg IV; may repeat in 30 minutes) and nifedipine (10 to 20 mg tid) are coronary and systemic vasodilator agents that are used for anginal pain caused by coronary artery vasospasm (e.g., Prinzmetal's angina), or atherosclerotic heart disease (ASHD).

Antiplatelet Agents

Antiplatelet agents such as aspirin (two tablets tid), dipyridamole (Persantin) (50 mg tid) and sulfinpyrazone (Anturane) (200 mg qd to qid), are sometimes used, since platelet aggregation is thought to play a significant part in decreasing coronary artery blood flow.

Nonoperative Dilatation of Coronary Artery Stenosis

Dilatation is sometimes employed in patients with single-vessel disease and a short history of pain. Its long-term usefulness, however, is still under investigation.

Coronary Artery Bypass Graft (CABG)

This procedure is indicated if a medical regimen fails and angina pain significantly interferes with the patient's ability to manage the activities of daily living. Approximately 60 per cent of patients who undergo coronary artery bypass grafting for incapacitating angina (with good left ventricular function) attain complete relief from pain, and an additional 20 per cent achieve partial relief. Although the risk of surgery has decreased dramatically during the past decade, the operative mortality rate still ranges from 0 to 3.5 per cent, depending on the number of coronary arteries involved and the state of the patient's left ventricular function.

Identification and Alteration of Manageable Risk Factors

Control of risk factors plays an important role in prevention and management of coronary artery disease.

Sympathetic and Attentive Listening

Listening to the patient talk about pain and its impact on lifestyle is advised. Determining the events that precipitate anginal attacks and helping the patient find creative solutions to these problems are indicated. It also should be emphasized to the patient that the occurrence of anginal pain does not necessarily mean he or she will definitely have an infarction.

—————— Myocardial Infarction ——————

GENERAL CONSIDERATIONS

Definition

Myocardial infarction (MI) is death (coagulative necrosis) of myocardial tissue resulting from an acute decrease in coronary blood flow or an abrupt rise in myocardial oxygen demand without sufficient coronary artery perfusion.

Classification

Anteroseptal MI. This involves a portion of the anterior wall as well as the intraventricular septum and results from occlusion of the left anterior descending artery.

Anterolateral MI. This type of MI involves a portion of the anterior as well as a portion of the lateral wall of the left ventricle and results from occlusion of the left circumflex artery.

Inferior (Diaphragmatic) MI. This involves the inferior portion of the left ventricle and is usually a result of right coronary artery occlusion.

Posterior MI. This involves the posterior portion of the left ventricle and can occur from either right coronary or circumflex artery occlusion.

Right Ventricular MI. This kind of MI is usually associated with right coronary artery occlusion. It is difficult to diagnose.

ETIOLOGY

Precipitating factors for MI are the same as those listed for angina pectoris. Causes of myocardial hypoperfusion and MI can be grouped according to intrinsic and extrinsic factors.

Intrinsic Factors

Coronary atherosclerosis with resultant thrombosis and occlusion is the underlying cause in nearly all MI. Less common causes (less than 10 per cent) include coronary embolism, vasospasm and inflammation. The last-named is more prevalent in younger individuals.

Extrinsic Factors

Decreased coronary artery perfusion can occur secondary to the effects of maximum compression on the subendocardium during systole. Coronary hypoperfusion may also result from severe hypotension or rapid ventricular rates with a significant decrease in diastolic filling time.

PATHOPHYSIOLOGY

Cellular Changes

Persistent ischemia (20 minutes to 2 hours) will produce irreversible cellular damage. Hypoxic cells are forced to find alternative energy substrates. Unable to use free fatty acids, the predominant energy source under normal aerobic conditions, myocardial cells must rely on anaerobic glycogenolysis. Unfortunately, anaerobic metabolism of glucose is a much less efficient means of energy production. As energy availability falls, metabolites accumulate, pH falls and myocardial function fails. This results in reduced myocardial contractility, decreased stroke volume, diminished ejection fraction, increased left ventricular end-diastolic pressure and altered ventricular wall compliance. Peripheral vascular resistance usually increases in response to the inevitable catecholamine release and tends to produce a greater central blood volume, increasing the workload of the ailing heart.

Zones of Infarction

A center core of *coagulative necrosis* occurs, in which all cells are dead, including myocardial cells, connective tissue and capillaries. This central area of necrosis is surrounded by potentially viable areas of *injury* and *ischemia* (see Fig. 11–6). Severely ischemic tissue may progress to necrosis if interventions are not implemented. By 24 to 96 hours after

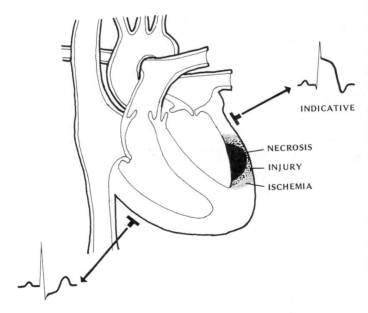

INDICATIVE

NECROSIS
INJURY
ISCHEMIA

RECIPROCAL

Figure 11–6.   Zone of transmural myocardial infarction with indicative and reciprocal ECG changes.

MI, there may be a significant increase in collateral blood flow to revitalize the ischemic area.

Extent of Infarction—Involvement of Myocardium

Myocardial Infarction.   MI can be divided into two major types.

Transmural Infarction.   This involves the full thickness of the myocardium from endocardium to epicardium (Fig. 11–6).

Subendocardial Infarction.   This is generally confined to the area of the subendocardium (Fig. 11–7).

Severity of Damage.   The amount of damage is dependent upon a number of different factors:

    a. Degree of coronary artery occlusion.
    b. Size and location of the area supplied by the narrowed vessels.
    c. Oxygen needs of the poorly perfused myocardium.
    d. Extent of collateral blood vessel development. (An occluded artery need not result in MI if there is extensive collateral circulation present.)

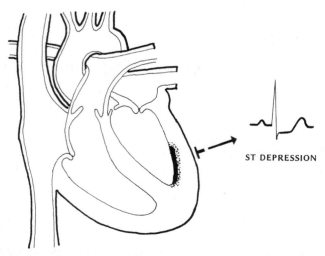

ST DEPRESSION

Figure 11–7.   Subendocardial infarction and ECG change.

Morphologic Changes

1. In the first 12 hours, the damaged myocardial tissue appears normal upon gross inspection.
2. In 18 to 48 hours, the infarcted tissue appears pale with focal, red-purple areas of interfiber hemorrhage.
3. In 2 to 10 days, the necrotic area is very apparent. The tissue appears yellowish and soft and contains areas of hemorrhage. This is the most likely time for ventricular rupture.
4. Within 10 days to 6 weeks, the necrotic tissue is replaced by gray, fibrous, noncontractile scar tissue.
5. In 2 months, the maximum density of scar tissue is achieved.

PATIENT ASSESSMENT

The diagnosis of myocardial infarction is based on the triad of the patient's clinical picture, the cardiac enzyme values and the electrocardiogram. Any of these factors, combined or alone, may be the basis for positive findings of myocardial tissue damage. (See Chapters 1, 2 and 3.)

Clinical Picture

The patient's clinical presentation will vary according to the size and location of MI and the individual's pre-infarction condition.

Pain. Although pain is a dramatic characteristic of MI, approximately 25 per cent of infarcts are unrecognized because the patient experiences very little or no discomfort. The following, however, are more typical findings.

Location. The pain is usually left precordial or substernal and radiates down the left arm, down both arms, or to the jaw, teeth, back or epigastric area.

Quality. The quality of pain is often described as crushing, gripping, stabbing, aching, constricting, numbing, viselike or like a heavy weight on the chest.

Duration. The chest pain of MI persists constantly for 20 minutes or longer.

Intensity. The pain is variable, often described as 5 or more on a rating scale of 1 to 10.

Precipitating Factors. The pain occurs during exertion or at rest. Myocardial infarction pain may awaken one from sleep.

Alleviating Factors. The pain of MI is not relieved by rest, position change or nitroglycerin. The use of opiates, particularly morphine sulfate, usually relieves the pain, but persistent discomfort may remain for hours.

General Appearance. The MI patient usually appears very anxious, weak, dyspneic, diaphoretic and restless, often moving about in the bed in an effort to find a position of comfort. Nausea and vomiting are common and may be due to severe pain, vagal stimulation or decreased cardiac output. Appearance may vary according to the location of MI. For example, patients with inferior MI tend to present with bradycardia, more gastrointestinal distress and hiccoughs.

Blood Pressure. Hypotension can occur secondary to a decrease in cardiac output or from beta-adrenergic stimulation (vasodilation) in response to severe pain.

Pulse. The pulse may be fast, slow, or irregular and often is weak and thready.

Temperature. Temperature may rise within 24 hours and may last 3 to 7 days, ranging from 37.5° to 38.8°C (100 to 101°F); it correlates with the extent of myocardial tissue damage.

Heart Rhythm. Heart rhythm is usually normal sinus rhythm (NSR). The potential for the occurrence of dysrhythmias is high during the first 24 hours after infarct.

Heart Sounds. Heart sounds are often muffled. S_3 and S_4 gallops indicating ventricular dysfunction may be present. Murmurs, not previously documented, may signify papillary muscle dysfunction. A friction rub, heard days to weeks after MI, heralds the presence of pericarditis.

Lung Sounds. Pulmonary rales indicating left ventricular failure may be noted in the lungs.

Apical Impulse (Point of Maximum Impulse, or PMI). Enlarged or laterally displaced impulses may occur transiently with MI. A normal impulse is located in the midclavicular, fifth intercostal space and should be no larger than 2 cm in diameter; it occurs as a brief, single impulse.

Skin.   Skin may be pale, cyanotic or mottled and often cool, clammy and moist owing to increased cardiac output and sympathetic discharge (increased peripheral vascular resistance).

Jugular Veins.   Increased distention may signify right ventricular failure. An early sign of left ventricular dysfunction is an increased amplitude of the "a" wave in the jugular vein.

Edema.   Ankle, pretibial and sacral edema are late indicators of heart failure.

Urinary Output.   This is often low, less than 20 ml per hour during the first 12 hours, but increases as cardiac performance improves.

Diagnostic Tests

ECG Changes.   Serial ECGs are usually needed to confirm the presence of infarction because the initial ECG may be normal or nonconclusive.
Indicative ECG Changes of Acute MI (see Fig. 11–6). Indicative changes involve abnormal findings in the leads facing the surface of the damaged area, including the following:
Pathological Q Wave.   The Q wave is 0.04 second or more in duration or is greater than 25 per cent of the R wave in depth, or both. The Q wave begins to develop within hours after the onset of MI. It is a permanent ECG pattern, representing irreversible transmural myocardial necrosis. The presence of a Q wave alone, without any supporting signs, may not be significant. However, a newly developed Q wave, even if it is narrow, may indicate infarction.
ST Segment Shift.   With *elevation,* there is a convex upward curvature. Usually, it is the earliest ECG finding of an impending MI. ST elevation represents reversible myocardial ischemic injury. It returns to the isoelectric line after a period of a few hours or days. In *depression,* a concave downward curvature is present. It may indicate ischemia or subendocardial infarction (see Fig. 11–7).
T Wave Inversion.   This indicates myocardial ischemia. When ischemia is alleviated, the T wave returns to an upright position. In patients with subendocardial infarction, the T wave is also inverted.
The Reciprocal ECG Changes of Acute MI (see Fig. 11–6).   Reciprocal changes involve findings in the leads facing

the opposite surface of the damaged areas, including the following:

a. No Q wave, but an increase in the height of the R wave.
b. Depressed ST segment.
c. Upright T wave.

Evolutional ECG Changes. The moment-to-moment changes of ST segment and T and Q waves during the course of MI indicate the progression of the condition. See Figure 11–8 for some typical changes.

Determination of MI Location. As listed in Table 11–1, the anatomical location of MI is determined by new findings of indicative or reciprocal ECG changes (or both) in the specific leads.

Enzymes. The diagnosis of MI often depends on the measurement of cardiac enzymes, especially when the ECG and clinical picture are not conclusive. Serial enzyme measurements, which are performed 6 to 12 hours apart are usually used for confirmation of MI. The most commonly used enzymes are listed in Table 11–2. For further details, please refer to Chapter 3.

Chest X-Ray. This is used to assess heart size and pulmonary vasculature.

Electrolytes. This study is used to assess hypo- or hyperkalemia and fluid balance.

Complete Blood Count (CBC). This rules out anemia and polycythemia. The white blood count (WBC) may rise to 14,000 per cubic millimeter or higher and reflects the extent of myocardial tissue damage.

Glucose. Glucose levels are used to test glucose metabolism. However, the intense adrenergic reaction to MI may transiently elevate blood sugar levels.

Blood Urea Nitrogen (BUN). This is used for assessing renal function and for adjusting drug dosages.

Triglyceride and Cholesterol Counts. These measurements rule out familial hyperlipidemia.

INDICATIVE
CHANGES

RECIPROCAL
CHANGES

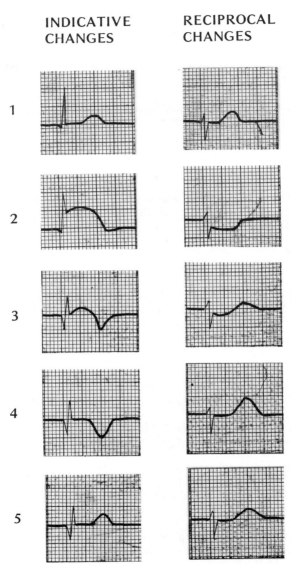

Figure 11–8. Evolutional ECG changes of MI. 1, Normal tracing; 2, hours after infarction; 3, few days after; 4, many days to weeks; 5, months to years.

Table 11–1.   DETERMINATION OF MI LOCATION

LOCATION OF MI	LEADS WITH INDICATIVE CHANGES	LEADS WITH RECIPROCAL CHANGES
Anteroseptal MI	V_1, V_2, V_3	II, III, AVF
Anterolateral MI	V_5, V_6, I, AVL	II, III, AVF
Inferior or diaphragmatic MI	II, III, AVF	I, AVL
Posterior MI (true)	III	V_1, V_2

Radioisotope Studies (Thallium Scan).   These studies assess the location and extent of MI.

Echocardiogram.   The echocardiogram evaluates heart size, configuration values and wall motion, hypokinesis, dyskinesis and akinesis.

Angiography.   Angiography usually demonstrates total obstruction or a high degree of stenosis.

ST Segment Mapping.   This procedure is used to predict myocardial necrosis.

COMPLICATIONS

Complications of MI

Arrhythmias.   Myocardial ischemia may cause many forms of arrhythmias and conduction defects. (See Chapter 12.)

Congestive Heart Failure.   MI is one of the major causes of congestive heart failure (CHF) (See Chapter 13.)

Cardiogenic Shock.   Infarction of 40 per cent or more of the myocardium usually leads to cardiogenic shock. This is one of the most severe complications of MI and is often fatal (See Chapter 14.)

Pericarditis.   Transmural MI often extends to the epicardial surface and causes inflammation. Diffuse pericarditis may lead to pericardial effusion. (See Chapter 16.)

Rupture of Papillary Muscles.   Rupture is usually caused by transmural MI and leads to sudden onset of mitral insufficiency and systolic murmur.

Table 11–2. COMMONLY USED CARDIAC ENZYMES

ENZYMES*	ISOENZYME†	ONSET OF ELEVATION	PEAK	RETURN TO NORMAL LEVEL
CPK	Yes (CK-MB)	6–12 hours	24 hours	3–4 days
SGOT	No	8–12 hours	36 hours	3–4 days
LDH	Yes	24–48 hours	3–6 days	8–14 days

*CPK, creatine phosphokinase; SGOT, serum glutamic-oxaloacetic transaminase; LDH, lactic dehydrogenase.
†CK-MB, creatine phosphokinase–MB.

Table 11–3. TREATMENT MODALITY RELATED TO MYOCARDIAL OXYGEN DEMANDS AND SUPPLY

↓ MYOCARDIAL OXYGEN DEMANDS	↑ MYOCARDIAL OXYGEN SUPPLY	OTHER
1. Bed rest	1. Oxygen administration	1. Corticosteroids
2. Sedation and pain relief	2. Antiarrhythmics	
3. Antipyretics	3. IABP	
4. Antiarrhythmics	4. Coronary artery streptokinase infusion	
5. Nitrates (sublingual, oral paste)	5. Coronary artery bypass graft	
6. Beta-blockers (propranolol, hadolol)	6. Hyaluronidase	
7. Intra-aortic balloon pump (IABP)	7. Nifedipine	
8. Calcium channel blockers (verapamil, nifedipine)		
9. Glucose-insulin-potassium, IV infusion		

Rupture of the Left Ventricle.   Extensive necrosis leads to thinness of the the left ventricular wall and to rupture. Hemopericardium, cardiac tamponade or death may follow.

Rupture of the Septum.   Left-to-right shunt occurs as a result of the rupture. The size of the shunt determines the extent of survival.

Ventricular Aneurysm.   The aneurysm is caused by over-stretching of a thin and noncontractile portion of the infarcted myocardium. It bulges with each systole and creates a prom-inent PMI. The paradoxical contraction leads to decreased cardiac output. It also leads to clot formation, which may cause systemic embolism. Ventricular aneurysm usually in-creases ventricular irritability as well.

Post–Myocardial Infarction Syndrome (Dressler's Syn-drome).   This syndrome consists of pericardial or pleural pain or both, malaise and fever. It usually begins 3 to 6 weeks after the onset of MI. The cause is presumably due to an autoimmune reaction to myocardial damage, affecting partic-ularly the pericardium, pleura and lungs.

Extension of MI.   It is caused by decreased cardiac output after MI and reduction of coronary artery blood flow to the injured myocardium.

Thromboembolism.   Mural thrombi often occur in associa-tion with extensive infarcts and in the presence of CHF.

Behavior Changes.   Denial, depression and overdependence are commonly observed among MI patients.

Treatment-Induced Complications
Complications Induced by Bed Rest

  a. Thromboembolism—those thrombi formed in the legs often lead to pulmonary embolism.
  b. Constipation.
  c. Depression and dependence.

Complications Induced by Medications
Hypotension.   This is often caused by analgesics (morphine sulfate), especially after repeated doses or in conjunction with the administration of nitrates. It can also be caused by

intravenous injection of cardiac depressants (quinidine, procainamide or phenytoin).

Hemorrhagic Pericardial Effusion.   This may be caused by
anticoagulant therapy.

Congestive Heart Failure.   Large doses of cardiac depressants (quinidine, procainamide, disopyramide, verapamil or
propranolol) may depress myocardial contractility.

Complications Induced by Invasive Procedures

Arrhythmias.   These are caused by irritation of the ventricles
by pacemaker electrodes or intracardiac catheters.

Subacute Endocarditis.   A pathogen could be introduced via
the invasive procedure.

Phlebitis.   This is caused by the irritation of the intravenous
catheter or of medication.

MEDICAL AND NURSING MANAGEMENT

Relief of Pain

Relief of pain is of primary importance. Intravenous morphine sulfate is the drug of choice. It is administered in
increments of 3 to 5 mg up to 20 mg or until the pain is
relieved. Should respiratory depression secondary to morphine sulfate administration occur, naloxone hydrochloride
(Narcan) may be given. Intravenous meperidine (Demerol),
in increments of 12.5 to 25 mg, is used if the patient
demonstrates hypersensitivity to morphine. Use of inhaled
nitrous oxide also appears to be effective. The use of nitrates
for the acute pain of myocardial infarction is often useful.
Intramuscular injections should be avoided, since they cause
an increase in total creatine phosphokinase (CPK) value.

Careful Monitoring

For early detection and treatment of complications, careful
monitoring is inherent to coronary care nursing. This includes
immediate recognition and treatment of life-threatening arrhythmias, as well as frequent physical assessment to ascertain
hemodynamic status. An elevated temperature should be
treated with acetaminophen (Tylenol), two tablets q 4 hours,
since the resultant tachycardia increases myocardial oxygen
demands. The presence of a "keep open" intravenous line

provides a direct route for administration of emergency medications.

Fear of Death

Allaying the patient's fear of death is of paramount importance. The sudden occurrence of severe chest pain and subsequent admission to the Coronary Care Unit have a profound emotional impact. Along with immediately administering analgesics, the nurse should demonstrate a calm, reassuring attitude. All procedures and restrictions and their purposes should be carefully explained to the patient and significant others. Sedation with diazepam (Valium), 5 to 10 mg qid, may be necessary.

Adequate Oxygenation

Adequate oxygenation should be maintained in all patients demonstrating hypoxemia. This may be accomplished via nasal prongs at a flow of 2 to 4 liters per minute. Administration of blood may be necessary if severe anemia is present.

Restriction of Physical Activity

A regimen of bed rest in a comfortable position, with commode privileges, is followed for the first 24 to 48 hours. Subsequent increases in the level of activity are dependent upon the patient's condition and tolerance. Passive exercise and antiemboli stockings aid in preventing phlebothrombosis.

Relief of Nausea and Vomiting

Nausea and vomiting should be relieved promptly, as they may result in vagal stimulation, leading to bradycardia and hypotension. Antiemetics, such as promethazine (Phenergan), 6 to 25 mg, may be administered intravenously every 6 hours as necessary.

Diet

Diet is usually restricted to liquids only for the first 24 hours. This decreases the risks of initiating nausea and vomiting, as well as diminishing the probability of aspiration, should cardiac arrest occur. After the first 24 hours, a soft diet, without added salt or caffeinated beverages, is taken. To aid in the determination of the patient's fluid status, intake and output or daily weight is measured routinely.

Stool Softeners

Stool softeners such as dioctyl sodium sulfosuccinate (Colace), one to two tablets qd, are employed on a routine basis to prevent straining and constipation.

Use of Anticoagulants

Anticoagulant use is controversial. In the absence of noted contraindications, the use of heparin in minidoses of 5000 units every 8 to 12 hours is thought to decrease the incidence of deep vein thrombosis after myocardial infarction.

Use of Antiplatelet Agents

The benefits of using antiplatelet agents are questionable.

Minimization of Ischemia and Infarcted Areas

Attempts to minimize ischemic and infarcted areas are currently being attempted via the methods listed in Table 11–3. Some of these methods are still controversial with regard to long-term benefits.

Sudden Cardiac Death

DEFINITION

Sudden cardiac death (SCD) is defined as death occurring within minutes to hours after the onset of a cardiac event.

ETIOLOGY

Ventricular fibrillation is the cause of SCD 98 per cent of the time. Other causes include asystole, heart block and bradycardia. Although the pathogenesis of SCD remains unknown, there is a high association with coronary artery disease. Cardiomyopathy, hypokalemia, myocarditis and aortic stenosis have also been implicated.

PATHOPHYSIOLOGY

The pathological lesion most frequently associated with SCD is selective myocardial necrosis, also called myofibrillar degeneration. This is evidenced by randomly occurring patches that contain dead myocardial cells surrounded by viable interstitial cells, nerves and capillaries. This lesion differs from the coagulative necropathy of myocardial infarction, in which all of the cells in the area, including interstitial cells, die and the lesion is localized to an area supplied by a coronary artery. There is evidence that hypoxia and catecholamines cause selective myocardial cell necrosis. Therefore, sympathetic stimulation and stress are also implicated. The actual mechanism of provoking ventricular fibrillation is not clearly understood, although all of these agents have been shown to lower the threshold to ventricular fibrillation by changing the duration of the vulnerable period.

CLINICAL MANIFESTATIONS

Physical Signs and Symptoms

Although some patients complain of vague, prodromal symptoms, there is usually sudden, painless loss of consciousness, apnea and absence of pulse. Although there are no immediate symptoms preceding the event, approximately 80 per cent of patients who have SCD also have other cardiovascular symptoms and have visited a physician 1 month prior to the event.

Electrocardiogram Changes

When monitored, these patients are often found to be in ventricular fibrillation. A 12-lead resting ECG after countershock may show ST segment depression, T wave flattening or prolongation of the Q-T interval.

Enzyme Changes

Cardiopulmonary resuscitation and countershock can elevate serum cardiac enzymes, which precludes diagnosis by enzyme elevations. However, isoenzymes are usually not diagnostic for MI.

MANAGEMENT

The management of SCD includes postresuscitative care (see Chapter 20), prevention of recurrence and psychological support.

Prevention of Recurrence

Antiarrhythmic Prescription. Patients frequently prove refractory to commonly used antiarrhythmics and, therefore, require close monitoring of response to drug therapy. Subsequent hospitalizations or Holter monitoring may be necessary for dosage adjustment or change of medication.

Patient and Family Teaching. Compliance to the recommended medical regimen should be emphasized. The patient and family should be given information regarding medications and follow-up and emergency measures. Cardiopulmonary resuscitation (CPR) training of significant others is essential.

Psychological Support

The patient and family live with the constant threat of imminent death and therefore may require much emotional support.

SUGGESTED READINGS

Angina Pectoris

Arcebal, A. G., and Lemberg, L.: Angina pectoris in the absence of coronary artery disease. *Heart and Lung*, 9:728, 1980.

Braunwald, E.: *Heart Disease*. Philadelphia, W. B. Saunders, 1980.

Gruntzig, A. R., et al.: Nonoperative dilatation of coronary artery stenosis. *N. Engl. J. Med.*, 301:2, 1979.

Hurst, J. W.: *The Heart*. New York, McGraw-Hill, 1978.

Rahimtoola, S. H.: Coronary bypass surgery for chronic angina—1981, A perspective. *Circulation*, 65:225, 1982.

Rubenstein, E., and Federman, D.: *Scientific American Medicine: Cardiovascular Medicine*, Vol. I. New York, Scientific American, 1981.

Sokolow, M., and Mellroy, M.: *Clinical Cardiology*. Los Altos, Lange Medical Publications, 1979.

Myocardial Infarction

Braunwald, E.: *Heart Disease*. Philadelphia, W. B. Saunders, 1980.

Leeche, R., Entman, M., Harrison, D., and Eknoyan, G.: Use of cardioactive drugs in acute myocardial infarction. *Heart and Lung*, 5:44, 1976.

Oliver, M. F.: The metabolic response to a heart attack. *Heart and Lung*, 4:57–60, 1975.

Scalzi, C.: Nursing management of behavioral responses following an acute myocardial infarction. *Heart and Lung,* 2:62, 1973.

Sokolow, M., and Mellroy, M.: *Clinical Cardiology.* Los Altos, Lange Medical Publications, 1979.

Sudden Cardiac Death

Cowan, M. J.: Sudden cardiac death and selective myocardial cell necrosis. *Heart and Lung,* 8:559, 1979.

Lown, B.: Sudden cardiac death. The major challenge confronting contemporary cardiology. *Am. J. Cardiol.,* 43:313, 1979.

Reichenbach, D. D., and Moss, N. S.: Myocardial cell necrosis and sudden death in humans. *Circulation,* 52(Suppl. III):60, 1975.

12

CARDIAC RHYTHM DISTURBANCES

GENERAL CONSIDERATIONS

Cardiac rhythm disturbances refer to any changes or disruptions of the normal sinus rhythm. Causes include any factors that interfere with normal cardiac function—coronary ischemia, chamber enlargement, valvular disorders, autonomic influences and effects of drugs. The mechanisms for rhythm disturbances can be categorized into two abnormalities.

1. Abnormality in automaticity.
   a. Increased automaticity may initiate premature ectopic beats.
   b. Decreased automaticity may result in bradycardia or arrest, allowing a latent pacemaker to take over.
2. Abnormality in conduction—conduction defects result in blocks or re-entry tachycardias.

CLASSIFICATION

Cardiac rhythm disturbances can be classified according to the following.
1. *Anatomical location*
   a. Supraventricular rhythms originate in the sinus node, the AV junction or the atria.
   b. Ventricular rhythms originate in the ventricles.
   c. Conduction disturbances can occur anywhere in the conducting system, from the SA node to the Purkinje fibers.
2. *Rate*
   a. Tachycardia refers to a heart rate greater than 100 beats per minute. An increased rate shortens diastole, thus decreasing coronary artery perfusion and diastolic filling time.
   b. Bradycardia refers to a heart rate less than 60 beats per minute. Decreased rates reduce cardiac output and permit ectopic takeover.

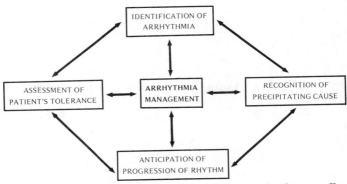

Figure 12–1. Interrelationship of nursing actions leading to effective arrhythmia management.

NURSING ACTION AND ARRHYTHMIA MANAGEMENT

In order to institute effective management, the coronary care nurse must be able to

1. Identify the arrhythmia.
2. Recognize the precipitating cause.
3. Anticipate the rhythm's progression.
4. Assess the patient's tolerance to the rhythm.

These actions are interrelated and may occur simultaneously, or their sequence may vary according to the clinical situation (see Fig. 12–1).

———————— Sinus Rhythms ————————

GENERAL CONSIDERATIONS

The function of the sinus node is under the continual influence of a sympathetic-parasympathetic counterbalance, attempting to maintain equilibrium within the body. Dysfunction of the sinus node most often occurs as a response to physiological and pathological stressors. It may also be altered by drugs, especially those that act through the autonomic nervous system.

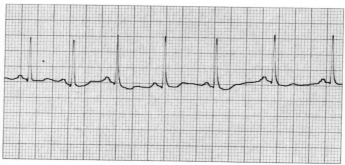

Figure 12–2. Sinus arrhythmia.

SINUS ARRHYTHMIA

ECG Criteria (see Figure 12–2)

Rate and Rhythm. The rate is 60 to 100 bpm*, and the rhythm is regularly irregular (cycle lengths vary by 0.12 second or more).

QRS Complex. This is usually normal.

P-Wave. This wave is upright in Lead II and is normal and constant in contour.

P-QRS Relationship. There is one P wave per QRS complex, and P precedes QRS with a PR interval of normal and constant duration.

Cause

Sinus arrhythmia is caused by a variation of rate in impulse formation due to the autonomic nervous system and pressure-volume reflexes within the heart and blood vessels.

Clinical Manifestations and Significance

An irregular pulse is auscultated. The patient is usually not aware of this arrhythmia, and it is often seen in healthy individuals.

---

*bpm—beats per minute.

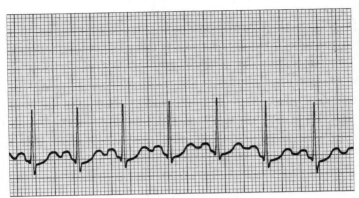

Figure 12–3. Sinus tachycardia.

Management

Usually, no treatment is indicated. If, however, the heart rate becomes too slow and the patient is symptomatic, the rate may be increased by exercise or administration of atropine, 0.5 to 1.0 mg intravenous (IV) push up to 2 mg.

SINUS TACHYCARDIA

ECG Criteria (see Figure 12–3)

Rate and Rhythm.   The rate is 100 to 150 bpm, and the rhythm is regular and starts and stops gradually.

QRS Complex.   This is usually normal.

P Wave.   This wave is upright in lead II and is normal and constant in contour; it may be buried in the preceding T wave.

P-QRS Relationship.   There is one P wave per QRS complex, and P precedes QRS with a P-R interval of normal and constant duration.

Cause

Sinus tachycardia results from an increase in rate of impulse formation due to normal and pathological stressors, including exercise, emotion, fever, pump failure, hyperthyroidism and certain drugs, including epinephrine, atropine, nitrates, isoproterenol, caffeine, nicotine and alcohol.

Clinical Manifestations and Significance

A rhythmically regular pulse between 100 and 150 bpm is auscultated. The rhythm responds to vagal stimulation by gradual slowing with subsequent return to specified tachycardiac rate when stimulation is withdrawn. This is a very common arrhythmia, its significance being related to the cause as well as to the patient's ability to tolerate an increase in heart rate. In a patient who has a myocardial infarction, sinus tachycardia at rest, in the absence of discernible stressors, may indicate a failing pump.

Management

Treat the underlying cause. Use of antipyretics, rest, sedation or withdrawal of offending drug may be indicated. If the condition is due to pump failure, management should follow what is described in Chapter 13.

SINUS BRADYCARDIA

ECG Criteria (see Figure 12–4)

Rate and Rhythm. The rate is less than 60 bpm, and the rhythm is regular.

QRS Complex. This is usually normal.

P Wave. The wave is upright in lead II and is normal and constant in contour.

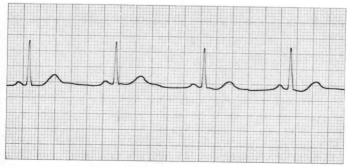

Figure 12–4. Sinus bradycardia.

P-QRS Relationship. There is one P wave per QRS complex, and P precedes QRS with a P-R interval of constant duration; the P-R may be slightly longer (0.22 second) than the normal limits.

Cause

Sinus bradycardia results from a decrease in the rate of impulse formation due to normal body responses to sleep, vagal stimulation or a well-conditioned athletic heart. It may also be due to pathological stressors such as decreased blood flow to the sinus node (as in diaphragmatic myocardial infarction), an oversensitive vagal response, increased intracranial pressure, hypothyroidism, hypothermia or depression. Drugs that may cause sinus bradycardia include beta-blockers, reserpine, digitalis and morphine.

Clinical Manifestations and Significance

A rhythmically regular pulse of less than 60 bpm is auscultated. The patient may be asymptomatic, especially if the occurrence of this rhythm is a normal physiological response. The patient becomes symptomatic only if the rate becomes slow enough to hinder adequate cardiac output, at which time syncope, angina or rapid ectopic rhythms may occur.

Management

Treatment is not indicated unless the patient becomes symptomatic. This rhythm usually is reversed by increasing sympathetic tone or decreasing vagal tone. The order of emergent intervention usually starts with atropine, 0.5 to 1 mg up to 2 mg given as an IV bolus. If atropine is ineffective, an isoproterenol (Isuprel) drip, with an average dose of 1 to 4 mcg per minute, may be initiated. If the bradycardia is resistant and the patient is symptomatic, pacemaker insertion is indicated.

SINUS BLOCK

First-Degree Sinus Block

This represents a delay in conduction between sinus node discharge and atrial depolarization that cannot be appreciated on the routine ECG.

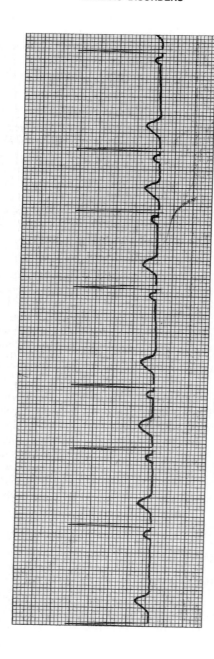

Figure 12–5. Sinus Wenckebach.

Second-Degree Sinus Block

There are two types of second-degree sinus block. Although their ECG criteria may vary, they are similar in cause, clinical manifestations and treatment.

Type I: Sinus Wenckebach
ECG Criteria (see Figure 12–5)

Rate and Rhythm. The rate is 60 to 100 bpm, and the rhythm is regularly irregular owing to a pause with an increase in sinus discharge after the pause.

QRS Complex. This is usually normal and is absent during pause.

P Wave. This wave is upright in lead II and is normal and constant in contour. It is absent during a pause. The P-P interval progressively shortens prior to a pause that is equal to less than two P-P intervals.

P-QRS Relationship. There is one P wave per QRS complex. P precedes QRS with a normal and constant P-R interval.

Type II: Sinus Exit Block Type II
ECG Criteria (see Figure 12–6)

Rate and Rhythm. The rate is 60 to 100 bpm, and the rhythm is regularly irregular due to a pause equal to an exact multiple of the cycle length (usually two times).

QRS Complex. This is usually normal and is absent during a pause.

P Wave. This wave is upright in lead II, and is normal and constant in contour. It is absent during a pause without loss of sinus cadence.

P-QRS Relationship. There is one P wave per QRS complex, and P precedes QRS with normal P-R interval.

Cause

Second-degree sinus block is caused by a dysfunction of sinus impulse conduction that results in an intermittent failure

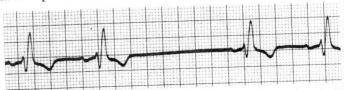

Figure 12–6. Sinus exit block, type II. (From Phillips, R. E., and Feeney, M. K.: *The Cardiac Rhythms*, 2nd ed. Philadelphia, W. B. Saunders, 1980, p. 94.)

to depolarize the atria. This may be due to an increase in vagal tone, disease of the conduction system, coronary artery disease involving the sinus node artery, acute infection or drugs (digitalis, salicylates, quinidine).

Clinical Manifestations and Significance

An irregular pulse is auscultated, the patient usually remaining otherwise asymptomatic. The significance depends upon the cause as well as the length of the pause. The most common cause of sinus Wenckebach is digitalis excess.

Management

Treatment is usually not warranted unless the patient becomes symptomatic and exhibits signs of decreased cardiac output. Determine and treat the underlying cause if possible. Otherwise, the nurse may need to use atropine, 0.5 to 1 mg as an IV bolus up to 2 mg; isoproterenol (Isuprel), 1 to 4 mcg per minute in IV drip; or a pacemaker, as the situation dictates.

Third-Degree Sinus Block

The terms "third-degree sinus block," "sinus arrest" and "atrial standstill" are sometimes considered synonymous. They will be discussed together in this chapter, as they all represent a cessation of sinus and atrial activity for an undeterminable amount of time and are manifested as well as managed in the same manner. Their main difference is in mechanism, sinus block being considered a failure in impulse conduction from the sinus node and sinus arrest being considered a failure in impulse formation in the sinus node. Both may result in atrial standstill.

ECG Criteria (see Figure 12–7)

Rate and Rhythm. When this block is present, the rate is 60 to 100 bpm, but the length of or frequency of the pause

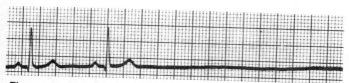

Figure 12–7. Third-degree sinus block. (From Phillips, R. E., and Feeney, M. K.: *The Cardiac Rhythms*, 2nd ed. Philadelphia, W. B. Saunders, 1980, p. 84.)

may result in the bradycardia range. The rhythm is irregular owing to a pause; it may or may not be an exact multiple of cycle length.

QRS complex.   This is usually normal; however, ventricular escape beats may be present.

P Wave.   This wave is upright in lead II, and is normal and constant in contour; it is absent during a pause.

P-QRS Relationship.   When the P wave is present, it precedes the QRS complex with a normal P-R interval. It may have an escape ectopic rhythm (ventricular) void of atrial activity.

Cause
Third-degree sinus block results from complete failure of sinus node impulse formation or extreme prolongation of its conduction time. This may be due to increased vagal stimulation, degenerative fibrosis or coronary artery disease involving the sinus node, inflammatory heart disease or drugs (digitalis or quinidine).

Clinical Manifestations and Significance
Depending upon the length of the pause, the patient will exhibit signs and symptoms ranging from a feeling that the heart has "skipped a beat" or "stopped momentarily" to angina to loss of consciousness. Atrial standstill may encourage a subordinate ectopic focus to take charge.

Management
Determine and treat the underlying cause. Although atropine, 0.5 to 1.0 mg IV bolus up to 2 mg, and isoproterenol (Isuprel) titrate, 1 to 4 mcg per minute in IV drip, may be of temporary benefit, a pacemaker is usually indicated if this rhythm is not tolerated.

SICK SINUS SYNDROME (Bradycardia-Tachycardia Syndrome)

ECG Criteria (see Figure 12–8)

Rate and Rhythm.   The rhythm is irregularly irregular, haphazardly varying between bradycardic and tachycardic ranges.

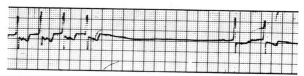

Figure 12–8. Sick sinus syndrome. (From Phillips, R. E., and Feeney, M. K.: *The Cardiac Rhythms*, 2nd ed. Philadelphia, W. B. Saunders, 1980, p. 87.)

QRS Complex. This is usually normal, although ventricular escape beats or aberrant beats may occur.

P Wave and P-QRS Relationship. These are dependent upon a variety of arrhythmias noted. Sick sinus syndrome first manifests itself electrocardiographically as a combination of various arrhythmias, including sinus arrest, sinus bradycardia, paroxysmal atrial tachycardia, atrial flutter, atrial fibrillation, junctional or ventricular escape rhythms, ventricular tachycardia and atrioventricular block. It also may be characterized by slow recovery time of the sinus node of 3 seconds or greater.

Cause

Sick sinus syndrome results from a dysfunction of the sinus node causing a decrease in rate or cessation of impulse formation or conduction usually due to myocardial infarction or degenerative fibrosis involving the sinus node, surgical trauma or inflammatory heart disease.

Clinical Manifestations and Significance

An irregularly irregular pulse may be auscultated, varying haphazardly from slow to rapid. Sick sinus syndrome most frequently occurs in the elderly, and depending upon its degree of severity, symptoms may be intermittent. The patient may be asymptomatic or may complain of palpitations, dizziness, shortness of breath, chest pain or syncope. He or she may present with congestive heart failure, Stokes-Adams attacks or cardiac arrest.

Management

If the patient is symptomatic, a pacemaker is indicated to prevent serious bradyarrhythmias and to allow for suppression of tachyarrhythmias.

———————— Atrial Rhythms ————————

GENERAL CONSIDERATIONS

Atrial arrhythmias arise when ectopic foci develop within the atrial walls owing to an increase in automaticity from various pharmacological, pathological and physical stimuli. When the rate of atrial ectopic depolarization exceeds that of the SA node, the atrial impulse pre-empts the normal sinus beat. The atrial focus then takes over the role of pacemaker for the heart.

ATRIAL PREMATURE BEATS (APBs)*

ECG Criteria (see Figure 12–9)

Rate and Rhythm. The rate is variable according to the frequency of extrasystoles. The rhythm is irregular owing to interruptions by the atrial extrasystoles, which are followed by incomplete compensatory pauses.

QRS Complex. This is usually normal and is similar in duration and contour to those appearing in the underlying rhythm.

P Wave. The P wave typically has a configuration different from that of the underlying sinus beat.

P-QRS Relationship. One P wave precedes each QRS complex in a 1:1 ratio. However, should the APB occur early enough in the cycle, its P wave may be buried in the preceding T wave, altering the T-wave contour. The P-R interval of the APB may vary from that of the underlying sinus beat.

———————

*Also called premature atrial contraction (PAC).

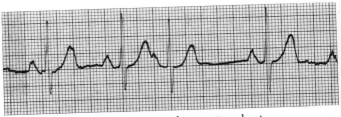

Figure 12–9. Atrial premature beat.

Cause

The atrial focus releases an impulse before the next normal firing of the sinoatrial (SA) node. The impulse depolarizes the atria, the SA node and the ventricles. Because of early depolarization, the SA node must then "reset" its rate, leading to the incomplete compensatory pause seen following most APBs.

Atrial premature beats are seen in normal individuals and are often precipitated by anxiety, ingestion of stimulants (e.g., caffeine), atrial dilation, organic heart disease, alcohol and smoking.

Clinical Manifestations and Significance

Atrial premature beats can be detected at bedside by palpation and auscultation but may be difficult to differentiate from premature ventricular beats. The patient may complain of "missed beats" or palpitations as the next normally occurring beat, following the APB, has a greater stroke volume and force of contraction.

Atrial premature beats are usually benign but, when seen in high frequencies (more than 6 bpm), may herald increasing atrial irritability and impending atrial fibrillation. They may also be indicative of early congestive heart failure (CHF).

Management

No treatment is usually necessary. Focus of therapy is directed toward treating the underlying cause. At times digitalis (following digitalization a maintenance dose of 0.125 mg to 0.5 mg daily), quinidine 200 to 400 mg q 6 to 8 hours or procainamide 250 to 500 mg q 3 to 4 hours may be used.

BLOCKED ATRIAL PREMATURE BEATS

ECG Criteria (see Figure 12–10)

The ECG criterion is the same as that for APBs, except that the premature P waves are not followed by QRS complexes. They appear as "dropped beats."

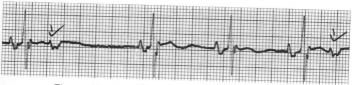

Figure 12–10. Blocked atrial premature beat.

Cause

The atrial focus releases an impulse before the normal firing of the SA node. If it occurs too early in the cycle, the impulse reaches the ventricles at a time when they are refractory to depolarization. As a result, the depolarization wave spreads through the atrium and is "blocked" at the AV node.

The causes are similar to those of regular ABPs. Digitalis excess may also induce this phenomenon.

Clinical Manifestations and Significance

These, too, are similar to those of APBs. If occurring with greater frequency, cardiac output may fall, and the patient may complain of "lightheadedness."

Management

Treatment is the same as for APBs.

WANDERING ATRIAL PACEMAKER (WAP)

ECG Criteria (see Figure 12–11)

Rate and Rhythm. The rate is 60 to 100 bpm, and the rhythm may be slightly irregular.

QRS Complex. This is usually normal.

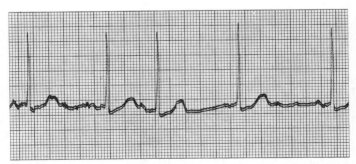

Figure 12–11. Wandering atrial pacemaker. (From Phillips, R. E., and Feeney, M. K.: *The Cardiac Rhythms*, 2nd ed. Philadelphia, W. B. Saunders, 1980, p. 102.)

P Wave. This wave is of variable configuration representing different foci. At least three different P wave configurations must be present for the diagnosis to be made.

P-QRS Relationship. One P wave precedes every QRS. The P-R interval may vary.

Cause

The focus randomly wanders about the atrium with impulses originating from the SA node, various atrial foci and the AV junction. It may result from enhanced vagal tone, digitalis excess or acute rheumatic fever.

Clinical Manifestations and Significance

The arrhythmia may occur in normal individuals. Its presence often goes unnoticed. There is little clinical significance unless the rate slows excessively.

Management

Usually no treatment is required. Digitalis may be held back if toxicity is suspected. If the rate slows excessively, atropine, 0.5 to 1.0 mg IV push up to 2 mg, may be given.

MULTIFOCAL ATRIAL TACHYCARDIA (MAT)*

---

*Also called chaotic atrial tachycardia (CAT).

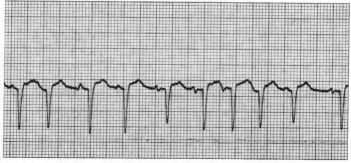

Figure 12–12. Multifocal atrial tachycardia.

ECG Criteria (see Figure 12–12)

The ECG criteria are the same as those for wandering atrial pacemaker except that the rate is between 100 and 250 bpm. This arrhythmia is nonparoxysmal in nature.

Cause

As in wandering atrial pacemaker, the pacemaker "jumps" around the atrium from the SA node to atrial foci to AV junctional foci. The major cause of MAT is chronic obstructive lung disease. Other causes include coronary artery disease (CAD), anesthesia, sepsis, and (infrequently) digitalis toxicity.

Clinical Manifestations and Significance

The pulse is rapid and irregular and indistinguishable from atrial fibrillation at the bedside. The fast rate may precipitate CHF, angina and hypotension.

Management

It is important to treat the cause. Digitalis should be held back if it is suspect, or it may be given as treatment (after digitalization, with a maintenance dose of 0.125 to 0.5 mg qd). Propranolol (0.5 to 1 mg per minute up to 5 mg IV or 10 to 20 mg PO qid) may be given if there is no underlying pulmonary disease. Verapamil (5 to 10 mg) in a slow IV bolus may be tried as well.

PAROXYSMAL ATRIAL TACHYCARDIA (PAT)

ECG Criteria (see Figure 12–13)

Rate and Rhythm. The rate is 150 to 250 bpm. The rhythm is precisely regular and occurs in a paroxysmal fashion, starting and stopping abruptly.

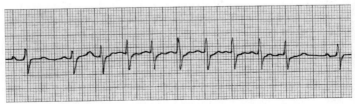

Figure 12–13. Paroxysmal atrial tachycardia.

QRS Complex. This is usually normal but may become aberrant if the rhythm persists.

P Wave. This wave is uniform throughout the duration of the arrhythmia. They may or may not be buried in the preceding T wave.

P-QRS Relationship. One P wave precedes each QRS.

Cause

Re-entry is the mechanism for this arrhythmia. It may occur in individuals with no evidence of heart disease. It often is precipitated by sympathetic nervous system stimulation, such as extreme emotions, caffeine ingestion, fatigue, smoking and excessive alcohol intake. Rheumatic heart disease, pulmonary emboli, thyrotoxicosis and cardiac surgery are less common causes.

Clinical Manifestations and Significance

With sudden onset, the patient may feel "rapid palpitations" and severe anxiety. This may be accompanied by angina, congestive heart failure (CHF) or shock secondary to a decrease in cardiac output and increased myocardial oxygen demand. It is the common arrhythmia associated with pre-excitation syndrome.

Management

Vagal stimulation from carotid sinus massage is particularly helpful in terminating PAT. Baroreceptor stimulation may also be initiated through the use of the Valsalva maneuver or vasopressors. Therapy may include use of digitalis (following digitalization, a maintenance dose of 0.125 to 0.5 mg qd), propranolol (0.5 to 1.0 mg per minute up to 5 mg IV or 10 to 20 mg PO qid), quinidine (200 to 400 mg PO q 6 hours), edrophonium (Tensilon, 10 mg IV over 30 seconds), and phenylephrine (Neo-Synephrine, 0.5 to 1.5 mg IV in 30 seconds, with blood pressure monitoring). Sedatives and tranquilizers can reduce sympathetic stimulation. Verapamil (5 to 10 mg slow IV push) has recently been proved to be the drug of choice for converting PAT to normal sinus rhythm. An oral dose of 80 to 160 mg·q8h can be used for preventing recurrence. Cardioversion is considered if these measures are ineffective.

PAROXYSMAL ATRIAL TACHYCARDIA WITH BLOCK

ECG Criteria (see Figure 12–14)

Rate and Rhythm. Atrial rhythm is precisely regular at a rate of 150 to 250 bpm. Because of varying degrees of AV block, the ventricular rate may or may not be regular and most often occurs at a rate of one half the atrial rate.

QRS Complex. This is usually normal but may broaden at higher rates.

P Waves. This wave often appears small and has a "snake-toothed" configuration.

P-QRS Relationship. There are two or more P waves for every QRS. The P-QRS relationship varies with the degree of AV block but is most often seen in a 2:1 ratio. The P-R interval is constant except in the instance of a "Wenkebach" type of block.

Cause

The mechanism is similar to that of PAT. It is, however, more often associated with organic heart disease and digitalis toxicity.

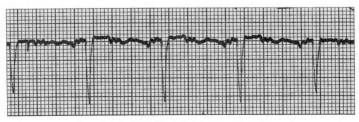

Figure 12–14. PAT with block.

Clinical Manifestations and Significance

This rhythm requires ECG monitoring for diagnosis. The clinical features resemble PAT. Cardiac output may fall, depending upon the rate and degree of block.

Management

Because digitalis toxicity is a significant contributor to this arrhythmia, it must be ruled out. If toxicity is present, the therapy is the same as for PAT, except that the drugs of choice include phenytoin (Dilantin, 50 mg IV q 5 minutes until control, up to 1000 mg) propranolol (0.5 to 1 mg per minute up to 5 mg IV, contraindicated if a high degree of block is present), and quinidine (200 to 400 mg q 6 hours), along with potassium supplementation.

ATRIAL FLUTTER

ECG Criteria (see Figure 12–15)

Rate and Rhythm.   The atrial rate is regular and usually greater than 300 bpm. The ventricular rate and rhythm, which may or may not be regular, depend upon the degree of AV block.

QRS Complex.   This is usually normal but may appear broadened as flutter waves become buried in the QRS.

P Wave.   These waves are replaced by "flutter waves," which are aberrant, and at high rates become bidirectional, demonstrating a characteristic "saw-toothed" pattern.

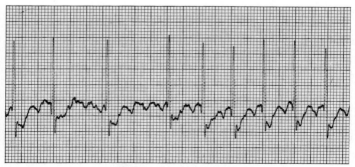

Figure 12–15.   Atrial flutter.

P-QRS Relationship. Typically, there are two or more flutter waves to every QRS complex. This ratio is highly variable and dependent on AV blocking. Most common are 2:1 and 4:1 blocks.

Cause

An atrial re-entry phenomenon is the underlying mechanism for this arrhythmia. Like PAT with block, the rapid waves of atrial depolarization are blocked at the AV node in varying ratios. This rhythm is most commonly found in the presence of organic disease such as coronary artery disease, mitral valve disease, hyperthyroidism or pulmonary embolism or may occur after cardiac surgery. It may also appear during bouts of atrial fibrillation following quinidine therapy.

Clinical Manifestations and Significance

The patient may not be aware of the arrhythmia except for sensing some "palpitations." Only in rapid ventricular rates (2:1 or 1:1 ratios) are symptoms of decreased cardiac output likely to be seen. Atrial flutter may be paroxysmal or chronic, and prognosis depends on the underlying disease process.

Management

Carotid sinus massage is useful only in temporarily slowing the ventricular response so that flutter waves can be identified. Drugs of choice include digitalis (maintenance dose of 0.125 to 0.5 mg qd) followed by quinidine (200 to 400 mg q 6 hours). Propranolol (0.5 to 1.0 mg IV not to exceed 5 mg or 10 to 40 mg PO qid) and procainamide (Pronestyl) (250 to 500 mg PO q 3 to 4 hours) may also be tried. Verapamil (5 to 10 mg slow IV push) has also been proved effective in controlling rapid ventricular rate. Cardioversion is always to be considered if pharmacological conversion fails (see Chapter 19). Atrial pacing may be attempted to capture the atria at a faster rate.

ATRIAL FIBRILLATION

ECG Criteria (see Figure 12–16)

Rate and Rhythm. The rhythm is highly irregular, with a ventricular rate ranging from less than 50 to more than 200. Any discernible atrial rate is greater than 350 bpm.

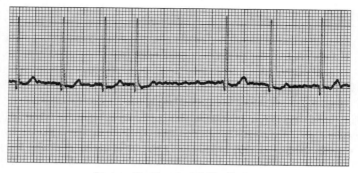

Figure 12–16.   Atrial fibrillation.

QRS Complex.   This is usually normal.

P Wave.   No P waves are discernible, and there is an irregular, undulating baseline.

P-QRS Relationship.   QRS complexes occur at irregular intervals in random association with the fibrillatory waves.

Cause

The atrial tissue can respond to impulses of more than 500 bpm. However, at the very rapid firing rates of an atrial ectopic focus, the entire atrium may not be able to recover from one depolarization wave when the next begins. This results in electrical and mechanical disorganization of the atria. The AV node is bombarded with impulses, most of which are blocked owing to the refractoriness of the AV node. Hence, the ventricular rhythm is very irregular.

Atrial fibrillation is common in older individuals. The causes are similar to those of atrial flutter and include restrictive pericarditis, atrial dilation, CHF and cor pulmonale.

Clinical Manifestations and Significance

The patient may be asymptomatic or may note palpitations and an irregular pulse. There is often a pulse deficit between apical and radial pulses. Because of atrial disorganization, there is no "atrial kick," which can decrease cardiac output by as much as 20 to 30 per cent. With increasing ventricular rates, cardiac output falls, resulting in shock, angina and CHF.

Mural thrombi formation is of concern, as blood may pool in the atria owing to inadequate emptying. This blood can clot, increasing the potential for pulmonary and cerebral vascular emboli.

Management

Treatment is the same as for atrial flutter. Anticoagulants may be given to decrease the threat of mural thrombi formation.

Junctional Rhythms (AV Nodal Rhythms)

GENERAL CONSIDERATIONS

Junctional rhythms occur as an escape mechanism or as an overdrive rhythm. They are usually classified as upper (AN, atrionodal), middle (N, nodal) and lower (NH, nodal His) as a convenient way of expressing the relationship of the P wave to the QRS complex.

JUNCTIONAL RHYTHM (Nodal rhythm, junctional or nodal escape beats)

ECG Criteria (see Figures 12–17, 12–18 and 12–19)

Rate and Rhythm.   The rate is 40 to 60 bpm, and the rhythm is regular.

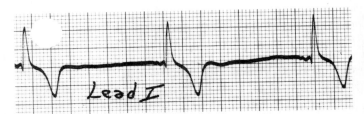

Figure 12–17.   Upper junctional rhythm. (From Phillips, R. E., and Feeney, M. K.: *The Cardiac Rhythms*, 2nd ed. Philadelphia, W. B. Saunders, 1980, p. 209.)

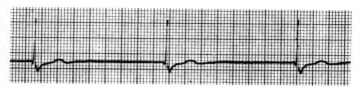

Figure 12–18. Middle junctional rhythm. (From Phillips, R. E., and Feeney, M. K.: *The Cardiac Rhythms*, 2nd ed. Philadelphia, W. B. Saunders, 1980, p. 209.)

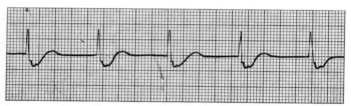

Figure 12–19. Lower junctional rhythm.

QRS Complex. This is usually normal.

P Wave. This wave is inverted in leads II, III, and AVF; it is abnormal in configuration and may not be visible (N origin).

P-QRS Relationship. There is one P wave per QRS complex. P may precede QRS (upper node, AN origin), may be hidden in QRS (middle nodal) or may follow QRS (lower, NH origin). PR depends upon the origin of impulse in the junction; when P precedes QRS, the P-R interval is shorter than normal, i.e., less than 0.12 seconds.

Cause

Junctional rhythm occurs as an escape mechanism when the sinus node is suppressed. This may be due to the effects of digitalis, coronary artery disease, carotid sinus massage or inflammatory heart disease.

Clinical Manifestations and Significance

A regular bradycardic pulse is auscultated. The patient must be monitored to differentiate the type of bradycardia present. This rhythm is a safety mechanism and is often transient. The patient remains asymptomatic unless the heart rate is sufficiently slow to cause inadequate cardiac output or to stimulate an irritable site outside the junction to take over, resulting in a tachyarrhythmia.

Management

Treatment is usually not indicated. Check for digitalis excess. If the slow heart rate is not tolerated, atropine, 0.5 to 1.0 mg up to 2 mg in an IV bolus, may be tried. If atropine is ineffective, the normal progression to isoproterenol drip, 1 to 4 mcg per minute or pacemaker or both is indicated.

JUNCTIONAL PREMATURE BEATS (JPBs)*

ECG Criteria (see Figure 12–20)

Rate and Rhythm. The rate is variable, depending upon the frequency of JPBs. The rhythm is irregular owing to the occurrence of premature beats, usually associated with an incomplete compensatory pause.

QRS. This is usually normal.

P Wave. This wave is as in junctional rhythm.

P-QRS Relationship. This relationship is as in junctional rhythm.

Cause

The underlying mechanism is increased automaticity of the AV junction, causing it to fire before the normal firing time

---

*Also called premature nodal contractions (PNC) and premature junctional contractions (PJC).

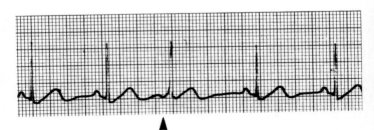

Figure 12–20. Junctional premature beat. (From Phillips, R. E., and Feeney, M. K.: *The Cardiac Rhythms*, 2nd ed. Philadelphia, W. B. Saunders, 1980.)

of the sinus node. This is usually due to ischemia of the junction or digitalis excess.

Clinical Manifestations and Significance

An irregular rhythm is auscultated that is difficult to differentiate from the occurrence of APBs without a monitor. JPBs usually are not noticed by the patient, although he or she may complain of a feeling that the "heart has skipped a beat." The occurrence of JPBs is not very common and is usually of little significance. However, if they occur frequently (more than six per minute), they reflect an increase in junctional irritability.

Management

Usually, treatment is not indicated. If JPBs are frequent, consider digitalis excess as a possible cause.

NONPAROXYSMAL JUNCTIONAL TACHYCARDIA (NPJT)

ECG Criteria (see Figure 12–21)

Rate and Rhythm. The rate is 65 to 130 bpm, and the rhythm is regular and starts and stops gradually.

QRS Complex. This is usually normal.

P Wave. The P wave is as in junctional rhythm.

P-QRS Relationship. This relationship is as in junctional rhythm.

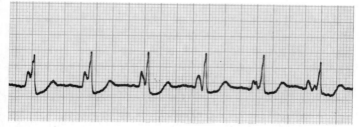

Figure 12–21. Nonparoxysmal junctional tachycardia competing with sinus rhythm.

Cause

The underlying mechanism is accelerated automaticity originating in the AV junction. It usually is a result of digitalis toxicity but may also be due to ischemia of the junctional tissue, myocarditis or cardiac surgery.

Clinical Manifestations and Significance

A regular pulse in the stated range is auscultated. The patient is usually asymptomatic owing to the range of the rate. However, he or she may show signs of inadequate cardiac output if the underlying condition does not tolerate increased rate or loss of atrial kick. Occurrence of this rhythm often indicates digitalis excess. In the patient with an underlying rhythm of atrial fibrillation, NPJT may be recognized as a slowing and regularization of the ventricular rate and is considered to be an early sign of digitalis toxicity. NPJT may also lead to AV dissociation.

Management

Treatment is usually not indicated. Consider digitalis excess. Carotid sinus massage will temporarily slow the rate but will not terminate this arrhythmia.

PAROXYSMAL JUNCTIONAL TACHYCARDIA (PJT)

ECG Criteria (see Figure 12–22)

Rate and Rhythm.   The rate is 140 to 250 bpm, and the rhythm is regular and starts and stops abruptly.

QRS Complex.   This is usually normal.

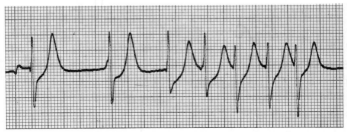

Figure 12–22.   Paroxysmal junctional tachycardia.

P Wave. This wave is as in junctional rhythm.

P-QRS Relationship. This relationship is as in junctional rhythm.

Cause

PJT is a re-entry tachycardia originating in the AV junction and is due to ischemia of the junctional tissue, left ventricular failure, inflammatory heart disease, thyrotoxicosis, emotional stress, coffee ingestion, smoking or digitalis excess.

Clinical Manifestations and Significance

A regular rapid pulse is auscultated. PJT often cannot be differentiated from PAT by ECG. It may be confused with ventricular tachycardia if bundle branch block is present, and it may occur in an individual without heart disease. If the increased heart rate or loss of atrial kick is not tolerated, the patient may exhibit signs of inadequate cardiac output.

Management

This arrhythmia usually is self limiting. Treatment is the same as for paroxysmal atrial tachycardia.

─────── Ventricular Rhythms ───────

GENERAL CONSIDERATIONS

Ventricular rhythms appear as either escape or overdrive (reentry) rhythms. They have more ominous significance than atrial or junctional rhythms.

IDIOVENTRICULAR RHYTHM (ESCAPE)

ECG Criteria (see Figure 12–23)

Rate and Rhythm. The rate is 20 to 40 bpm (inherent rate of ventricles), and the rhythm is regular.

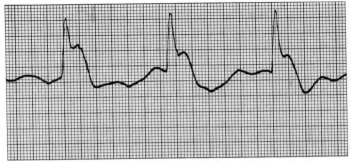

Figure 12–23. Idioventricular rhythm.

QRS Complex. The QRS is wide, greater than 0.11 second, and appears bizarre, with the T wave opposite the terminal portion of the QRS complex.

P Wave. This may or may not be present.

P-QRS Relationship. If P waves are present, they have no relationship to the QRS complexes.

Cause

Idioventricular rhythms result when there is failure of impulse formation or blockage of conduction from higher pacemaker centers. The ventricle assumes control by default. The ventricular pacemaker is located in the ventricular wall or the septum, below the bundle of His bifurcation.

Clinical Manifestations

Symptomatology depends on the patient's tolerance of the slow rate. The patient may experience signs of decreased cardiac output and usually has no activity tolerance. It is clinically significant because the patient's life is totally dependent upon this only remaining pacemaker.

Management

As idioventricular rhythm represents the only remaining escape mechanism, it should not be suppressed with lidocaine. Although the ventricles are often refractory to atropine,

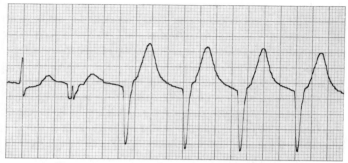

Figure 12–24. Accelerated ventricular rhythm.

sometimes a response can be evoked from a higher pacemaker. Intravenous isoproteronol (1 to 4 mcg/min IV drip)
may increase the ventricular rate. Pacemaker insertion is
indicated if tolerance to the rhythm is poor.

ACCELERATED VENTRICULAR RHYTHM (AVR)*

ECG Criteria (see Figure 12–24)

Rate and Rhythm.   The rate is 60 to 100 bpm, and the
rhythm is regular.

QRS Complex.   The QRS is wide, greater than 0.11 second.
Fusion beats often occur. The complex occurs at regular
intervals with occasional retrograde P waves.

P-QRS Relationship.   There is no relationship between P-
QRS, as this is AV dissociation.

Cause

The cause of AVR is heart disease, most often acute
myocardial infarction or digitalis toxicity. The ventricular rate
exceeds the dominant rate and takes pacemaking control.

Clinical Manifestations and Significance

The arrhythmia is generally benign, as the patient is
asymptomatic. However, loss of atrial kick may precipitate
hypotension.

---

*Also called accelerated idioventricular rhythm (AIVR).

Management

The rhythm is usually not treated. Digitalis should be withheld, if toxicity is suspected. Monitor the patient for development of other, life-threatening arrhythmias. If the rhythm is initiated by an R-on-T phenomenon or is associated with ventricular tachycardia, lidocaine is used to suppress it.

VENTRICULAR PREMATURE BEATS (VPBs),* VENTRICULAR ECTOPY, VENTRICULAR EXTRASYSTOLE

There are many types of VPBs. They can be classified according to their location in the cycle, focus of origin, or frequency of occurrence.

Location in the Cycle

Early VPB

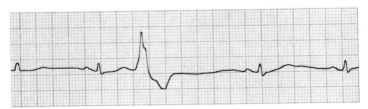

Figure 12–25.   Early VPB.

R-on-T VPB

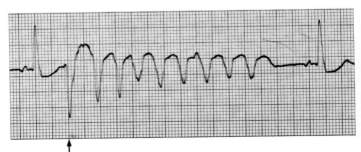

Figure 12–26.   R-on-T VPB—leads into ventricular tachycardia.

---

*Also called premature ventricular contractions (PVCs) and premature ventricular beats (PVBs).

Interpolated VBP

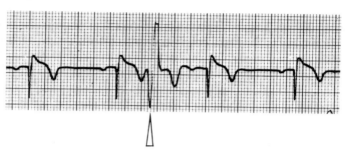

Figure 12–27. Interpolated VPB. (From Phillips, R. E., and Feeney, M. K.: *The Cardiac Rhythms*, 2nd ed. Philadelphia, W. B. Saunders, 1980, p. 262.)

Late VPB

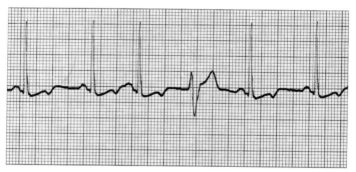

Figure 12–28.   Late VPB.

Focus of Origin
Unifocal VPBs

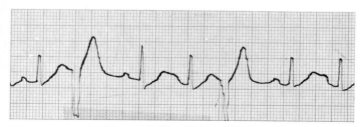

Figure 12–29.   Unifocal VPB.

Multifocal VPBs

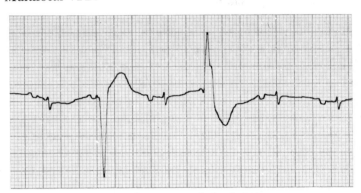

Figure 12–30.   Multifocal VPB.

Right VPBs

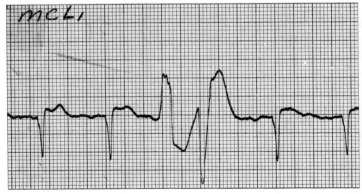

Figure 12–31.   Right VPB (fourth beat) preceded by a left VPB (third beat).

Left VPBs

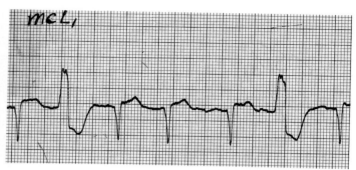

Figure 12–32. Left VPB.

Frequency of Occurrence

Isolated VPBs

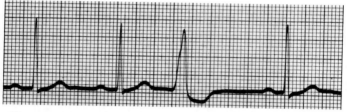

Figure 12–33. Isolated VPB. (From Phillips, R. E., and Feeney, M. K.: *The Cardiac Rhythms*, 2nd ed. Philadelphia, W. B. Saunders, 1980, p. 268.)

Bigeminy (VPB Occurs Every Other Beat)

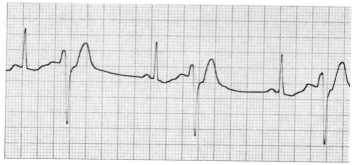

Figure 12–34. Ventricular bigeminy.

Trigeminy (VPB Occurs Every Third Beat)

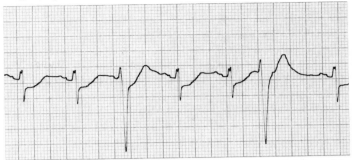

Figure 12–35. Ventricular trigeminy (first six beats) followed by ventricular bigeminy.

Quadrigeminy (VPB Occurs Every Fourth Beat)

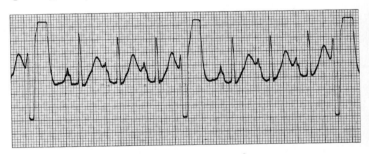

Figure 12–36. Ventricular quadrigeminy.

Paired VPBs (Two VPBs in a Row)

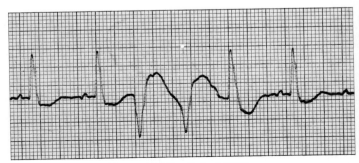

Figure 12–37. Paired VPBs.

ECG Criteria (see Figures 12–25 to 12–37)

Rate and Rhythm.   The overall rate is determined by the underlying rhythm. The rhythm is irregular owing to interruption by the VPBs, which are usually followed by complete, compensatory pauses.

QRS Complex.   The complex is wide (greater than 0.11 second), and appears bizarre. The configuration of the VPB will vary according to the site of origin. The T wave is in the opposite direction of the terminal portion of the QRS.

P Wave.   This wave is usually not visible.

P-QRS Relationship.   There is none.

Causes

The prematurity of VPBs signifies active pacemaking rather than an escape mechanism. The cause of VPBs can be anything that leads to enhanced ventricular automaticity. Causes include hypoxia, hypokalemia, acidosis, myocardial infarction, fiber stretch due to volume overload or heart failure, toxic agents such as digitalis, beta stimulants such as aminophylline, increased myocardial workload due to exercise or high metabolic states and mechanical irritation from pacemaker malfunction and intracardiac catheters.

Clinical Manifestations and Significance

Early diastolic VPBs are more ominous than those occurring later in the cycle. R-on-T phenomena pose the greatest threat owing to the their proximity to the heart's vulnerable period; ventricular tachycardia and ventricular fibrillation may be triggered. Multifocal VPBs indicate increased ventricular irritability and are considered more serious than unifocal beats. Also of great concern are VPBs that occur with increasing frequency or in pairs. Ventricular bigeminy often indicates digitalis excess.

Management

1. In an acute myocardial infarction, initial treatment should be directed at suppression of the VPBs. When VPBs occur at a rate of greater than six per minute, or greater than 10 per cent of the heart rate, a bolus of intravenous lidocaine

(50 to 100 mg IV bolus) should be given and followed by continuous intravenous infusion (2 to 4 mg per minute).

2. Other myocardial depressants used include procainamide (100 to 200 mg IV bolus slowly, followed by 1 to 4 mg per minute of IV drip), quinidine (200 to 400 mg q 6 hours), propranolol (10 to 40 mg qid), phenytoin (50 mg q 5 minutes not to exceed 1000 mg), and disopyramide (300 mg initially followed by 100 to 200 mg PO q 6 hours).

3. Treatment includes the elimination of provoking causes, when possible. This may include discontinuation of digitalis; correction of hypoxia, acidosis and electrolyte imbalances (especially potassium); limitation of exercise; and volume unloading.

4. Atropine is given if the VPBs are occurring secondary to bradycardia (0.5 to 1 mg IV push up to 2 mg).

VENTRICULAR TACHYCARDIA (VT)

Definition

Ventricular tachycardia is defined as three or more sequential VPBs at a rate of greater than 100 per minute.

ECG Criteria (see Figure 12–38)

Rate and Rhythm. The rate is 100 to 250 bpm, usually 130 to 170. The rhythm is slightly irregular.

QRS Complex. This is wide, greater than 0.11 second. Fusion and capture beats may be present.

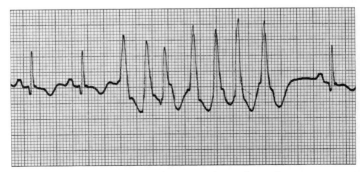

Figure 12–38. Ventricular tachycardia.

P Wave. This may be noted at regular intervals, as the atria usually remain under the control of the SA node. Occasional retrograde P waves may be noted.

P-QRS Relationship. There is usually none because of the AV dissociation. However, retrograde conduction may capture the atria and produce retrograde P waves.

Cause

All factors that cause ventricular ectopy can cause tachycardia, although it is most commonly caused by myocardial infarction. The irritable focus fires repetitively until it spontaneously ceases or therapy intervenes. The repetitive discharge is usually a result of a re-entry mechanism within the ventricular myocardium.

Clinical Manifestations and Significance

Ventricular tachycardia is ominous, as it can deteriorate into ventricular fibrillation. The clinical features vary with the rate and duration. Long, fast tachycardias are usually not tolerated by the patient and produce symptoms of decreased cardiac output and cerebral hypoperfusion. Ventricular tachycardia can be mimicked by supraventricular tachycardias, but vagal stimulation affects supraventricular tachycardia (SVT) and not VT and, therefore, is an important differentiation.

Management

Choice of treatment is related to the rate and tolerance of the rhythm.

1. Tachycardias causing loss of consciousness must be terminated immediately with electroshock therapy. A precordial thump may terminate the rhythm and can be tried while charging the defibrillator.
2. Lidocaine boluses of 75 to 100 mg are given for less threatening tachycardias and are followed by continuous intravenous drips at 2 to 4 mg per minute.
3. When ventricular tachycardia proves refractory to lidocaine, alternative pharmacological agents are procainamide (Pronestyl), 100 to 200 mg IV bolus slowly, followed by 1 to 4 mg per minute of IV drip; bretylium (Bretylol), 5 to 10 mg/kg, slowly repeated in 15 to 30 minutes and then q

6 hours or IV drip at 1 to 2 mg per minute; phenytoin (Dilantin), 100 to 200 mg IV q 5 minutes, not to exceed 1000 mg; propranolol (Inderal), 0.5 to 1 mg IV up to 5 mg; quinidine, 16 mg per minute IV bolus until control is reached but before toxicity occurs; and potassium replacement.

4. Ventricular pacing may override the rhythm and allow return of control to the sinus node.
5. Surgery is sometimes performed to resect aneurysms or site of origin of ectopy.
6. The best treatment of VT is prevention, ranging from the use of a prophylactic lidocaine drip to interventions that decrease myocardial oxygen demands.

VENTRICULAR FLUTTER

ECG Criteria (see Figure 12–39)

Rate and Rhythm.   The rate is 150 to 300 bpm with regular oscillations.

QRS Complex.   The complex resembles a wound coil being pulled apart; no distinct QRS complexes are present.

P Wave.   There is none present.

P-QRS Relationship.   None.

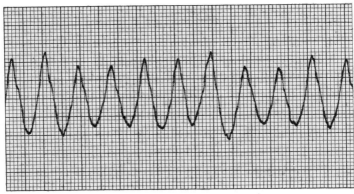

Figure 12–39.   Ventricular flutter.

Cause

Underlying causes are hypoxia, R-on-T phenomenon, myocardial infarction, drug toxicity and irritation from intracardiac catheters.

Clinical Manifestations and Significance

Ventricular flutter is a transition stage between ventricular tachycardia and ventricular fibrillation. If not treated, it is fatal in 3 to 5 minutes. The patient is pulseless and apneic and has no auscultated heartbeat.

Management

Immediate electroshock therapy at 200 to 400 joules (watt-seconds) and cardiopulmonary resuscitation (CPR) should be initiated to maintain circulation.

VENTRICULAR FIBRILLATION

ECG Criteria (see Figure 12–40)

There are irregular undulations of different shapes and amplitude. No distinct QRS, ST segments or T waves can be seen. Ventricular fibrillation is described as being coarse or fine.

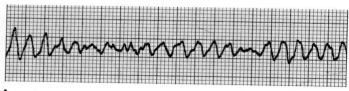

A

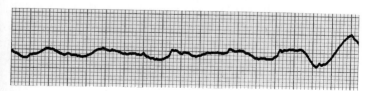

B

Figure 12–40. Ventricular fibrillation. *A*, Fine. *B*, Coarse.

Cause

It is associated with coronary artery disease, acute myocardial infarction (MI), advanced heart block, R-on-T phenomenon, digitalis or quinidine toxicities, hypoxia, hypothermia, electric shock and sudden death syndrome. The ventricles quiver, with erratic electrical discharges in every direction. The electrical discharges do not produce contractions.

Clinical Manifestations and Significance

There is no pulse, the patient is apneic and cardiac standstill occurs. There is loss of consciousness and sometimes seizures if cerebral anoxia persists.

Management

Immediate treatment is electroshock therapy with 200 to 400 joules (watt-seconds). CPR is initiated to maintain circulation. Epinephrine (10 ml of 1:1000 via IC or IV) is sometimes used for fine ventricular fibrillation to increase responsiveness to electroshock therapy.

VENTRICULAR ASYSTOLE

ECG Criteria (see Figure 12–41)

The monitor shows a straight line or P waves without any QRS.

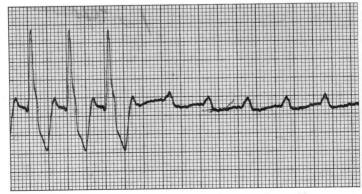

Figure 12–41. Ventricular asystole.

Cause

There is complete suppression of ventricular response.

Clinical Manifestations and Significance

The patient is pulseless, apneic and moribund.

Management

Initiate CPR immediately. Isoproterenol (2 ml of 1:5000 IV or IC), epinephrine (10 ml of 1:1000 IV, IC or intratracheal) or calcium chloride ($CaCl_2$, 5 to 10 ml of 10 per cent solution) given intravenously may aid in restoration of electrical activity. Pacing may also be tried.

AGONAL RHYTHM

ECG Criteria (see Figure 12–42)

The rate is very slow, with wide, "sloppy" QRSs. No P waves are seen.

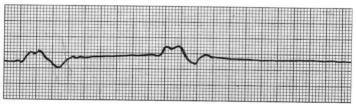

Figure 12–42.   Agonal rhythm.

Cause

Agonal rhythm represents the heart's feeble attempt to maintain electrical activity in the phase of cellular death.

Clinical Manifestations and Significance

The patient is pulseless, apneic and moribund.

Management

The patient usually does not respond to treatment.

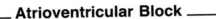

_____ Atrioventricular Block _____

GENERAL CONSIDERATIONS

Atrioventricular block is a rhythm disturbance caused by conduction impairment located in any site of the AV node, bundle of His and bundle branches. This disturbance delays or prevents the sinus impulse from reaching the ventricles. It may be transient or permanent, incomplete or complete. According to the severity of the disturbance, AV blocks can be classified as first, second or third degree.

FIRST-DEGREE AV BLOCK

ECG Criteria (see Figure 12–43)

Rate and Rhythm.   The atrial and ventricular rates, 60 to 100 bpm, are the same, and the rhythms are regular.

QRS Complex.   The QRS is normal.

P Wave.   The P wave is normal.

P-QRS Relationship.   One P wave precedes each QRS. The P-R interval is prolonged, more than 0.20 second.

Cause

The mechanism of prolonged P-R interval is merely the delaying of impulse propagation or the prolonging of conduction time in the AV node. Ischemia of the AV node, congenital anomalies, rheumatic fever and excessive vagal influence (effects of digitalis) are the common causes of first-degree AV block.

Clinical Manifestations and Significance

First-degree AV block is the least severe of the three forms. Patients are asymptomatic. The only clinical finding may be a soft first heart sound.

Management

First-degree AV block usually requires no therapy except for treating the underlying causes. Monitor carefully for possible progression to advanced degrees in patients with myocardial infarctions, though this is unlikely.

SECOND-DEGREE AV BLOCK

Second-degree AV block has two forms: Type I (Wenckebach or Mobitz Type I) and Type II (Mobitz Type II). The ECG features and clinical significance are quite different for each. However, both forms are characterized by intermittent dropped QRS complexes.

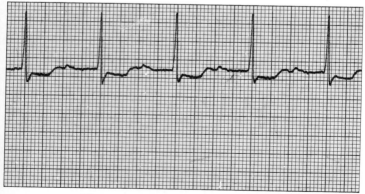

Figure 12–43.   First-degree AV block.

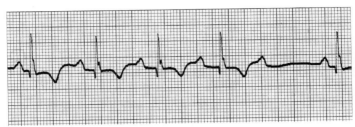

Figure 12–44. Second-degree AV block, Mobitz Type I.

Second-Degree AV Block—Wenckebach or Mobitz Type I

ECG Criteria (see Figure 12–44)

Rate and Rhythm. Five observations can be made.

1. Atrial rate is greater than ventricular rate. Both are between 60 and 100 bpm.
2. Atrial rhythm is regular; ventricular rhythm is irregular.
3. The R-R intervals become progressively shorter until one QRS is dropped, and then the longest R-R interval occurs. This cycle repeats.
4. Each cycle may consist of a group of two to six QRS complexes.
5. The longest R-R interval is less than twice the length of the shortest R-R interval.

QRS Complex. This is normal but is dropped periodically.

P Wave. The P wave is normal.

P-QRS Relationship. One P wave precedes each QRS except the last P wave of each cycle. The P-R interval of each succeeding beat in the cycle is progressively prolonged.

Cause

His bundle recording has demonstrated that this type of AV block usually is due to delaying conduction in the AV node and proximal to the bundle of His. It is often caused by digitalis toxicity, myocardial infarction or acute rheumatic fever.

Clinical Manifestations and Significance

Second-degree AV block, Mobitz Type I, usually causes no symptoms because the ventricular rate is adequately maintained. Occasionally, clinicians may recognize the first heart sound becoming progressively softer with intermittent pauses. Its diagnosis, however, is dependent on the characteristic ECG criteria. It may progress to complete AV block, particularly in the elderly.

Management

No treatment is indicated as long as the ventricular rate is adequate for perfusion. Therapy is usually directed toward eliminating the underlying causes, such as stopping digitalis, treating infection and so on. Occasionally, a temporary pacemaker may be used. Monitor for possible progression to a higher degree of block. Atropine, 0.5 to 1 mg, IV bolus, up to 2 mg, may be used temporarily for a low rate that is not tolerated well.

Second-Degree AV Block—Mobitz Type II

ECG Criteria (see Figure 12–45)

Rate and Rhythm.   Four observations may be made.

1. Atrial rate may vary from bradycardia to tachycardia but is usually between 60 and 100 bpm.
2. Ventricular rate depends on the grade of blocks present (2:1, 3:1, 4:1 or 3:2).
3. Atrial rhythm is regular.
4. Ventricular rhythm may be regular or regularly irregular.

QRS Complex.   The QRS is normal.

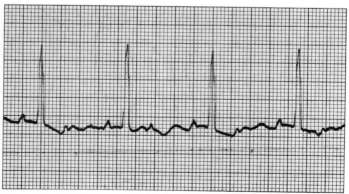

Figure 12–45.   Second-degree AV block, Mobitz Type II.

P Wave.　This wave is normal.

P-QRS Relationship.　Each QRS is preceded by a P wave, but not all P waves are conducted. Therefore, the P to QRS ratio may be 2:1, 3:1, 4:1 or 3:2. The P-R interval of conducted beats may be normal or prolonged, but they are always constant.

Cause
Second-degree AV block, Mobitz Type II—is usually caused by myocardial infarction, other organic heart disease and digitalis intoxication. In diaphragmatic myocardial infarction (DMI), the conduction defect is usually in the AV node owing to right coronary artery involvement. In anterior myocardial infarction (AMI), the disturbance is usually located in bundle branches because of left coronary artery involvement.

Clinical Manifestations and Significance
Patients are usually asymptomatic unless the ventricular rate is extremely low. They may feel dizzy or weak or may show other signs of low cardiac output. Mobitz Type II is considered more serious than Mobitz Type I AV block. The prognosis of Type II AV block is better when associated with DMI than AMI. In DMI, the block is often reversible, whereas in AMI it tends to advance to complete AV block.

Management
Treatment should be directed toward alleviation of the underlying causes, including withholding cardiac depressant medications. Temporary and permanent pacemaker insertions are often indicated for Mobitz Type II second-degree AV block. If a pacemaker is not immediately available, isoproterenol IV drip (titrate, 1 to 4 mcg per minute) may be used to maintain a heart rate that renders adequate cardiac output. Atropine may be tried in an attempt to increase inherent rate.

THIRD-DEGREE AV BLOCK (COMPLETE HEART BLOCK)

ECG Criteria (see Figures 12–46 and 12–47)

Rate and Rhythm.　Five observations can be made.

1. Atrial rate ranges from 60 to 100 bpm.
2. Ventricular rate ranges from 20 to 40 bpm if activated by

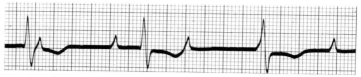

Figure 12–46. Third-degree AV block with ventricular escape. (From Phillips, R. E., and Feeney, M. K.: *The Cardiac Rhythms*, 2nd ed. Philadelphia, W. B. Saunders, 1980, p. 210.)

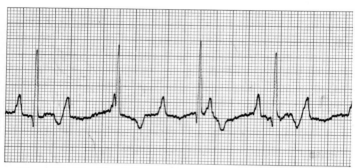

Figure 12–47. Third-degree AV block with junctional escape.

a ventricular pacemaker; it ranges from 40 to 60 bpm if activated by a junctional pacemaker.
3. Atrial rhythm (P-P interval) is regular.
4. Ventricular rhythm (R-R interval) is regular.
5. P-P intervals are not equal to R-R intervals.

QRS Complex. Two points can be noted.

1. The complex is normal, if activated by a junctional pacemaker.
2. The complex is greater than 0.11 second, if activated by ventricular pacemaker.

P Wave. This is normal.

P-QRS Relationship. There is none; atria and ventricles are independently depolarized by two separate pacemakers. Third-degree AV block is one form of AV dissociation.

Cause

Third-degree heart block can be caused by coronary artery disease, degenerative fibrosis of the conducting system, surgery, congenital anomalies, trauma, myocarditis and drug toxicity (digitalis, procainamide, quinidine and verapamil). Although the site of block may occur in the AV node (QRS is normal), more often it is located in the bundle branches (QRS is wide).

Clinical Manifestations and Significance

Patients may experience hypotension, angina and signs of CHF when the heart rate drops to 20 to 40 per minute (symptomatic bradycardia). Sudden ventricular asystole may accompany third-degree AV block. Together, they produce Stokes-Adams syndrome, loss of consciousness and even death. Low ventricular rate may also precipitate premature ventricular ectopies and tachyarrhythmias. However, in some patients, when third-degree AV block is not associated with acute myocardial infarction, it can be tolerated without symptoms.

Management

Sudden development of third-degree AV block in MI patients presents a clinical emergency. CPR may be necessary in conjunction with other modes of therapy. If a temporary pacemaker is not immediately available, isoproterenol (titrate, 1 to 4 mcg per minute) IV drip or atropine (0.5 up to 2 mg) IV push may be used to maintain ventricular rate until a pacemaker can be inserted. Permanent pacemaker implantation is indicated for irreversible third-degree AV block with symptoms.

＿＿ Intraventricular Conduction Defects ＿＿

GENERAL CONSIDERATIONS

Definition

Conduction impairments occur at any location of the conducting system distal to the His bundle. They may lead to third degree (complete) A-V block.

Types

1. Right bundle branch block (RBBB).
2. Left bundle branch block (LBBB).
3. Left anterior hemiblock (LAH).
4. Left posterior hemiblock (LPH).
5. Bifascicular block occurs when RBBB coexists with either LAH or LPH.
6. Trifascicular block occurs when RBBB coexists with both LAH and LPH.

QRS Morphology

The QRS usually becomes wider owing to the alteration of ventricular activation sequence.

RIGHT BUNDLE BRANCH BLOCK (RBBB)

ECG Criteria (see Figure 12–48)

Rate and Rhythm.   These depend on the patient's basic rate and rhythm. However, they are always sinus or supraventricular in origin.

QRS Complex.   This is equal to or more than 0.12 second.

P Wave.   This is usually normal if present.

P-QRS Relationship.   This relationship is dependent upon the underlying rhythm, i.e., sinus versus atrial fibrillation.

12-Lead ECG.   There is a wide R or R′ in V_1 and a wide S wave in I, V_5 and V_6.

Cause

1. In RBBB the supraventricular impulse is delayed or blocked in the right bundle branch.
2. The sequence of ventricular depolarization is
   a. Septal activation from left to right first.
   b. Left ventricular depolarization second.
   c. Right ventricular depolarization last.
3. The common causes of RBBB are coronary artery disease, right ventricular hypertrophy and acute pulmonary emboli.

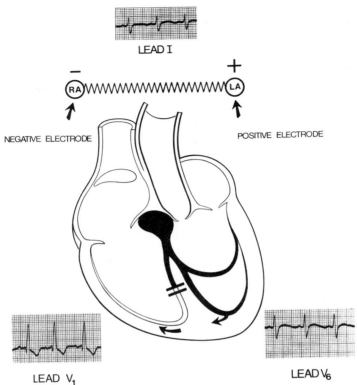

Figure 12–48. Right bundle branch block. (From Phillips, R. E., and Feeney, M. K.: *The Cardiac Rhythms*, 2nd ed. Philadelphia, W. B. Saunders, 1980, p. 241.)

Clinical Manifestation and Significance

1. RBBB enhances the split of the second heart sound due to the discrepancy of activation time in the two ventricles.
2. RBBB often coexists with a hemiblock or hemiblocks in MI patients. These patients may develop complete AV block and have angina and ventricular arrhythmias.
3. RBBB pattern often represents ventricular aberrance due to a prolonged refractory period of the RBB.

Management

Medical treatment is focused on the underlying cause. A pacemaker may be inserted in MI patients who develop bifascicular or trifascicular block. Recognition of the RBBB pattern often helps the CCU nurse to differentiate ventricular aberrance from ectopy.

LEFT BUNDLE BRANCH BLOCK (LBBB)

ECG Criteria (see Figure 12–49)

The ECG criteria are the same as these for RBBB except

1. The QRS is often wider, between 0.14 and 0.16 second.
2. On 12-lead ECG, there is
   a. A wide notched R in I, AVL and V_6.
   b. rS or QS in V_1.

Cause

1. In LBBB, the supraventricular impulse is delayed or blocked at the left main bundle.
2. The sequence of ventricular depolarization is
   a. Septal activation from right to left first.

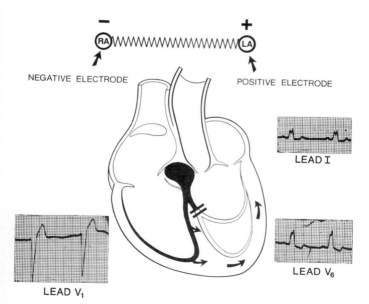

Figure 12–49.   Left bundle branch block. (From Phillips, R. E., and Feeney, M. K.: *The Cardiac Rhythms*, 2nd ed. Philadelphia, W. B. Saunders, 1980, p. 238.)

   b. Right ventricular depolarization second.

   c. Left ventricular depolarization last.

3. LBBB is commonly a result of coronary artery disease involving a large segment of the left ventricle. It may also occur in degenerative diseases and left ventricular hypertrophic disorders.

Clinical Manifestations and Significance

1. Clinical manifestation is dependent on the underlying disorders or on the presence of associated arrhythmias.

2. A paradoxical split of the second heart sound may be present owing to the alteration of ventricular activation sequence.

3. LBBB makes diagnosis of MI difficult because it changes the direction of septal activation and obliterates both the normal and the pathological Q waves on ECG.

Management

Medical treatment is focused on the underlying disease. Close observation for clinical progression to advanced AV block should be applied for acute MI patients with LBBB.

LEFT ANTERIOR HEMIBLOCK (LAH)

ECG Criteria (see Figure 12–50)

The ECG criteria are the same as those for BBB except

1. The QRS duration is within normal limits.

2. On 12-lead ECG:

   a. Left axis deviation is greater than −30 degrees.

   b. q is in I.

   c. r is in II, III and AVF.

Cause

1. The impulse is delayed or blocked at the left anterior fascicle of the left bundle.

2. The sequence of the left ventricular depolarization is

   a. The posterior and inferior portion first.

   b. The anterior and superior portion last.

3. The causes are similar to those of LBBB.

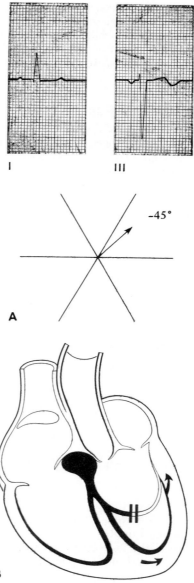

Figure 12–50. Left anterior hemiblock. *A*, ECG changes and axis. *B*, Diagram of heart. (*B* from Phillips, R. E., and Feeney, M. K.: *The Cardiac Rhythms*, 2nd ed. Philadelphia, W. B. Saunders, 1980, p. 249.)

Clinical Manifestation

The patient with LAH is asymptomatic. It is the most common form of hemiblock. Clinically, it often coexists with RBBB in patients with septal infarction.

Management

No particular treatment is indicated. General management is directed toward the underlying cause.

LEFT POSTERIOR HEMIBLOCK (LPH)

ECG Criteria (see Figure 12–51)

The ECG criteria are the same as those for LAH except on 12-lead ECG:

1. Right axis deviation of + 120 degrees or more.
2. r in I.
3. q in II, III and AVF.

Cause

1. The lesion of impulse blockage is in the posterior fascicle of the left bundle branch.
2. The sequence of the left ventricular depolarization is
   a. The anterior and superior portion first.
   b. The posterior and inferior portion last.
3. The causes are similar to those of LBBB.

Clinical Manifestation and Significance

Although the patient with LPH is asymptomatic, LPH often indicates widespread left ventricular disease. LPH may also coexist with RBBB. As a result, complete AV block may develop.

Management

No treatment is indicated unless it is associated with other clinical signs and symptoms. A pacemaker may be inserted if LPH coexists with RBBB.

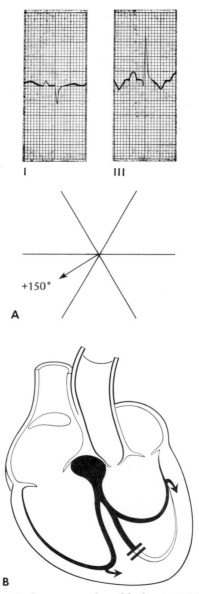

Figure 12–51. Left posterior hemiblock. *A*, ECG changes and axis. *B*, Diagram of heart. (*B* from Phillips, R. E., and Feeney, M. K.: *The Cardiac Rhythms*, 2nd ed. Philadelphia, W. B. Saunders, 1980, p. 250.)

ABERRANT CONDUCTION

Definition

Aberrant conduction is defined as abnormal ventricular conduction of a supraventricular impulse, resulting in a wide, deformed QRS complex.

Cause

1. Intraventricular conduction defects.
2. Anomalous pathway conduction.
3. Premature supraventricular impulse that reaches the ventricles before they are fully repolarized.

Significance

Aberrant conduction is often confused with ventricular ectopy. This may result in inappropriate rhythm management.

Criteria Commonly Used for Identifying Aberrance

1. Definite P-QRS relationship: If the underlying rhythm has a normal or constant P-QRS relationship, so will the aberrantly conducted rhythm.
2. Triphasic rsR' in V_1 or qRS in V_6: Aberrance often resembles RBBB patterns because the right bundle takes a longer time to repolarize (see Fig. 12–52).
3. Early cycle premature beat after a long R-R interval: When the heart rate is slow, ventricular repolarization also tends to be slow. Therefore, an early cycle premature supraventricular beat may fall during the incomplete refractory period of the ventricles.

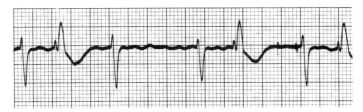

Figure 12–52. Aberrance of RBBB pattern. (From Phillips, R. E., and Feeney, M. K.: *The Cardiac Rhythms*, 2nd ed. Philadelphia, W. B. Saunders, 1980, p. 245.)

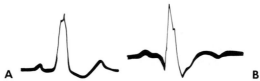

Figure 12–53. *A*, Taller right "rabbit ear" pattern. *B*, Taller left "rabbit ear" pattern.

4. Absence of compensatory pause: Aberrant premature beats usually reset the sinus firing time and cause no compensatory pause.
5. Initial vectors of the aberrant and normal QRS are similar.
6. A wide QRS of taller right "rabbit ear" pattern may often represent aberrance, and a wide QRS of taller left "rabbit ear" pattern may often represent ventricular ectopy (see Fig. 12–53).

Pre-Excitation Syndrome

GENERAL CONSIDERATIONS

Definition

1. Pre-excitation occurs when a portion of the ventricle is activated early by a congenital or acquired accessory conducting pathway between the atrium and the ventricle, resulting in a delta wave (a slur) in the initial portion of the QRS and a short P-R interval.
2. Pre-excitation syndrome consists of the characteristic delta wave on ECG as well as clinical presentation of a superventricular tachyarrhythmia (PAT or atrial fibrillation).

Mechanism

1. The impulse through the accessory pathway reaches the ventricle early because it bypasses the normal delay in the AV node.
2. The PAT is thought to be initiated by an atrial premature

beat (APB), which precipitates a re-entry phenomenon between the normal and the accessory pathways.

3. The mechanism that produces atrial fibrillation is not clearly understood. However, fast ventricular response in atrial fibrillation is caused by the short refractory period of the accessory pathway.

Classification

The two most commonly described pre-excitation syndromes are

1. Wolff-Parkinson-White (WPW) syndrome.
2. Lown-Ganong-Levine (LGL) syndrome.

WOLFF-PARKINSON-WHITE (WPW) SYNDROME

ECG Criteria (see Figure 12–54)

Rate and Rhythm. The rhythm usually resembles normal sinus rhythm with a tendency for frequent tachyrhythmias.

QRS Complex. This is greater than 0.10 second with delta wave.

P Wave. The P wave is usually normal.

P-QRS Relationship. One P wave precedes one QRS. The P-R interval is less than 0.12 second.

Types. Electrocardiographically, WPW syndrome can be classified into the following types:
Type A: Delta wave is positive on V_1 through V_2.
Type B: Delta wave is negative on V_1 through V_2 or V_3 and positive on V_4 through V_6.

Cause

1. WPW syndrome can be caused by various congenital or acquired cardiac defects. It may be associated with mitral valve prolapse, Ebstein's anomaly of tricuspid valve, cardiomyopathy and septal defects.
2. The connecting pathways between atria and ventricles may be located posteriorly (Type A) in the left side (Kent bundle), anteriorly (Type B) in the right side or in the septal region of the heart. Only invasive electrophysiological studies can precisely determine the site or sites.

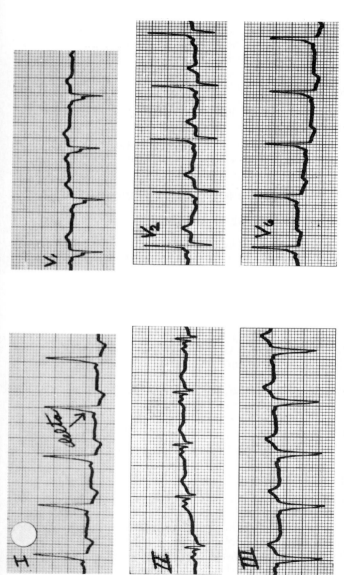

Figure 12–54. WPW syndrome. (From Phillips, R. E., and Feeney, M. K.: *The Cardiac Rhythms*, 2nd ed. Philadelphia, W. B. Saunders, 1980, pp. 171 and 172.)

Clinical Manifestations and Significance

WPW anomaly usually produces no signs or symptoms other than ECG criteria. When it is associated with supraventricular tachyrhythmias, PAT occurs more frequently than atrial fibrillation. The frequency and severity of the occurrence of tachyrhythmias determine the prognosis. Repetitive attacks can be disabling. Atrial fibrillation with rapid ventricular rate can cause ventricular fibrillation and sudden death.

Management

1. Medical therapy of patients with WPW syndrome is directly aimed toward preventing and controlling the PAT or atrial fibrillation or both.
2. Medications are used to suppress premature beats or to equalize the refractory periods of the normal and accessory pathways in order to discourage re-entry phenomenon. Propranolol, procainamide and quinidine may be used to accomplish this purpose.
3. The use of digitalis in WPW syndrome is still controversial.
4. If pharmacological means are ineffective, a pacemaker may be used to override the tachyrhythmia.
5. In markedly symptomatic patients, surgical intervention is indicated if the anomalous pathway can be determined.
6. Nursing management of PAT and atrial fibrillation is the same as discussed in the chapters on atrial dysrhythmias.

LOWN-GANONG-LEVING (LGL) SYNDROME

ECG Criteria

These are the same as described for WPW syndrome except that QRS duration is within normal limits (0.08 second).

Cause

1. LGL syndrome is a variant form of WPW syndrome.
2. The only difference is that the bypass responsible for LGL syndrome connects the atrium to the distal portion of the AV node (not the ventricle).
3. All impulses enter the bundle of His before the ventricles are activated. When the ventricles are depolarized in the normal manner, the QRS duration remains normal.

Clinical Manifestations and Significance

Patients with LGL syndrome may also experience palpitations and tachyrhythmias. Again, the prognosis depends on the frequency and severity of the attacks.

Management

The management is the same as for WPW syndrome.

SUGGESTED READINGS

Sinus Rhythms

Braunwald, E.: *Heart Disease*. Philadelphia, W. B. Saunders, 1980.

Chung, E. K.: Sick sinus syndrome: current views. In *Modern Concepts of Cardiovascular Disease*. Dallas, American Heart Association, 1980.

Hurst, J. W., et al.: *The Heart, Arteries and Veins*. New York, McGraw-Hill, 1978, pp. 644–646, 672–673, 677–682.

Phillips, R. E., and Feeney, M. K.: *The Cardiac Rhythms: A Systematic Approach to Interpretation*. 2nd ed. Philadelphia, W. B. Saunders, 1980, pp. 55–93.

Atrial Rhythms

Goldman, M.: *Principles of Clinical Electrocardiography*, 10th ed. Los Altos, Lange Medical Publications, 1979.

Phillips, R. E., and Feeney, M. K.: *The Cardiac Rhythms: A Systematic Approach to Interpretation*, 2nd ed. Philadelphia, W. B. Saunders, 1980.

Sokolow, M., and McIlroy, M.: *Clinical Cardiology*. Los Altos, Lange Medical Publications, 1979.

Junctional Rhythms

Braunwald, E.: *Heart Disease*. Philadelphia, W. B. Saunders, 1980, pp. 660–661.

Damato, A. N., and Lau, S. H.: His bundle rhythm. *Circulation*. 40:527, 1969.

Ventricular Rhythms

Goldman, M.: *Principles of Clinical Electrocardiography*, 10th ed. Los Altos, Lange Medical Publications, 1979.

Phillips, R. E., and Feeney, M. K.: *The Cardiac Rhythms: A Systematic Approach to Interpretation*, 2nd ed. Philadelphia, W. B. Saunders, 1980.

Sokolow, M., and McIlroy, M.: *Clinical Cardiology*. Los Altos, Lange Medical Publications, 1979.

Atrioventricular Block

Goldman, M. J.: *Principles of Clinical Electrocardiography*, 10th ed. Los Altos, Lange Medical Publications, 1979.

Kastor, J. A.: Atrioventricular block. *N. Engl. J. Med.*, 292:462, 1975.

Pelletire, G. B., and Marriott, H. J. L.: Atrioventricular block: Incidence in acute myocardial infarction and determinants of its degrees. *Heart and Lung*, 6:327, 1977.

Intraventricular Conduction Defects

Goldman, M. J.: *Principles of Clinical Electrocardiography*, 10th ed. Los Altos, Lange Medical Publications, 1979.

Phillips, R. E., and Feeney, M. K.: *The Cardiac Rhythms: a Systematic Approach to Interpretation*, 2nd ed. Philadelphia, W. B. Saunders, 1980.

Sweetwood, H. M., and Boak, J. G.: Aberrant conduction. *Heart and Lung*, 6:673, 1977.

Pre-Excitation Syndrome

Gallagher, J. J., et al.: The pre-excitation syndromes. *Progr. Cardiovasc. Dis.*, 20:285, 1978.

Papa, L. A., Saia, J. A., and Chung, E. K.: Ventricular fibrillation in Wolff-Parkinson-White syndrome, Type A. *Heart and Lung*, 7:1015, 1978.

Pritchett, E. L. C., and Gallagher, J. J.: Differential diagnosis and acute treatment of tachycardia with normal QRS morphology. *Prac. Cardiol.*, 4:84, 1978.

13

CONGESTIVE HEART FAILURE

GENERAL CONSIDERATIONS

Heart failure occurs when the heart fails to function as an effective pump. Congestion results in accumulation of blood in vascular beds and fluid in various parts of the body. Congestive heart failure (CHF) is often described as right sided or left sided, although failure in both sides may be present at the same time and one can progress to the other. In left-sided heart failure, fluid accumulates in the pulmonary venous circulation, whereas in right-sided heart failure, fluid accumulates in the systemic venous circulation. CHF can also be conceptualized according to the direction of the main force of blood flow. In forward failure, cardiac output is decreased. In backward failure, blood accumulates behind in one or both ventricles and the venous system. Clinical manifestations are dependent on the stage and progression of the heart failure.

ETIOLOGY

Any condition that interferes with the efficiency of the heart as a pump will eventually cause the heart to fail. The mechanism and conditions responsible for heart failure can be summarized as follows:

Decreased Myocardial Contractility

1. Coronary artery disease—ischemia, myocardial infarction (MI)
2. Pericardial tamponade
3. Ventricular aneurysm
4. Cardiomyopathy
5. Infiltrative diseases
   a. Myocarditis
   b. Amyloidosis
   c. Hemochromatosis
   d. Sarcoidosis
6. Collagen disorders
   a. Rheumatoid disorders
   b. Lupus
   c. Scleroderma

Excess Myocardial Workload

1. Increased afterload
   a. Hypertension
   b. Aortic or pulmonary stenosis
   c. Obstructive hypertrophic cardiomyopathy
   d. Chronic obstructive pulmonary disease—cor pulmonale
2. Increased preload
   a. Mitral, tricuspid valve insufficiency
   c. Aortic valve insufficiency
   c. Congenital left and right shunting
   d. Arrhythmia
3. Increased body demands
   a. Severe anemia
   b. Pregnancy
   c. Thyrotoxicosis
   d. Paget's disease
   e. Arteriovenous fistulas
   f. Nutritional deficiency (beriberi)

PATHOPHYSIOLOGY

Physiological Considerations

Function of the heart is indicated by its ability to maintain adequate blood supply to various parts of the body, not only during the resting state but also during physiological stress. The blood pumped out by the heart during each minute is called cardiac output. Cardiac output is the product of stroke volume times heart rate (CO = SV × HR). Heart rate is a primary cardiac reserve source for increasing cardiac output when stroke volume decreases. Stroke volume, the amount of blood ejected with each heartbeat, is determined by three major factors: preload, afterload and myocardial contractility.

Preload. This is the force or tension of the myocardium at the end of diastole or just before the onset of ventricular contraction. Clinically, it is represented by ventricular filling pressure. According to Frank-Starling's Law, the more the myocardial fibers are stretched (increased preload) up to a point, the stronger the myocardial contraction (increased stroke volume) will be. When the myocardium is stretched beyond that point, a reduction of cardiac output results.

Afterload. This refers to the total aortic pressure (imped-ance) that resists left ventricular ejection. Therefore, when the systemic arterial pressure increases, the work of the heart increases; when the systemic arterial pressure decreases, the work of the heart decreases.

Myocardial Contractility. This is the intrinsic ability of the myocardial fibers to shorten. For any given level of end-diastolic stretch (preload), an increase in stroke volume re-flects an increase in contractility; conversely, a decrease in stroke volume reflects a decrease in contractility.

Pathological Consequences (Fig. 13–1)

Forward Failure. One of the primary abnormalities in heart failure is reduction of myocardial contractility. In turn, the stroke volume decreases and cardiac output falls, regardless of the increase of heart rate. To compensate the reduced circulatory volume, the body activates the sympathetic nerv-ous system: the cardiac reserve mechanism. This activation leads to the following phenomena:

Increase in Heart Rate. In an attempt to balance the dimin-ished stroke volume and restore cardiac output, the heart rate increases. Besides the stroke volume, the amount of increase depends on the sympathetic response of the body.

Arteriolar Constriction. Reduction of blood flow to the kidneys, skin, splanchnic organs and skeletal muscles repre-sents an effort to maintain coronary and cerebral circulation.

Increase of Venous Tone. Facilitation of blood return to the heart from the periphery serves to enhance ventricular filling and to help maintain cardiac output.

Sodium and Water Retention. Reduced renal blood flow and renal arteriolar constriction trigger the renin-angiotensin mechanism, leading to increased aldosterone production and retention of sodium and water. The retained sodium and water increase venous volume returning to the heart, thus raising the ventricular filling pressure. A decrease in blood pressure also triggers the release of antidiuretic hormone, thus leading to further water retention.

Increased venous tone and sodium-water retention maxi-mize Frank-Starling's mechanism. However, in a failing heart,

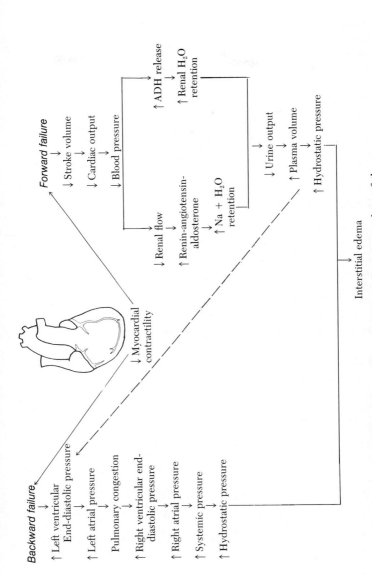

Figure 13–1. Pathophysiology of congestive heart failure.

they increase congestion and ventricular workload, further jeopardizing the myocardial contractility.

Backward Failure.   Backward failure may develop concurrently with forward failure, the degree of which is dependent on the acuity of the failing heart. As blood volume increases, the pulmonary hydrostatic pressure exceeds the pulmonary capillary colloid pressure, and the filtration pressure forces fluid into the interstitial space and alveoli. Consequently, pulmonary edema results. If the congestion accumulates over a longer period, the initially left-sided heart failure may progress to right-sided heart failure, causing systemic accumulation of fluid. Right-sided heart failure can also be caused by prolonged pulmonary hypertension.

PATIENT ASSESSMENT

Accurate assessment of the degree of congestion provides parameters for determining appropriate diuretic dosages. Evaluation of the heart as a pump reveals a need for selecting appropriate measures to maximize the pumping action. The effects of reduced cardiac output are evaluated in order to optimize nursing care planning.

Assessment includes correlation of patient history, physical assessment and diagnostic test results.

Patient History

Careful history-taking should identify subjective data and precipitating events that contributed to the need for hospitalization. Myocardial infarction is frequently a cause of CHF and should be explored.

Therefore, data collection should include the following:

1. Past history of cardiovascular disease, MI, hypertension, atherosclerotic heart disease, CHF, and treatment of CHF.
2. Pain, tightness or discomfort in the chest.
3. Increased episodes of shortness of breath with exertion over the last few days or weeks.
4. Activity intolerance, especially to normal daily activities.
5. Swelling noted in the ankles or lower legs.
6. Weight gain over the past few days.
7. Nocturnal pattern: the most comfortable degree of elevation for sleep and the number of times awakened with nocturnal dyspnea.

8. Current medications: diuretics and digitalis and adherence to prescribed regimen.
9. Diet: amount of sodium restriction and recent dietary indiscretions.
10. Recent systemic illness (e.g., pneumonia, anemia).
11. Recent increase of exertion.

Physical Assessment

Physical assessment of CHF includes recognition of signs and symptoms of CHF and underlying pathophysiology.

Signs and Symptoms of Decreased Cardiac Output
    a. Fatigue
    b. Increased heart rate
    c. Weak, thready pulse
    d. Narrow pulse pressure
    e. Hypotension
    f. Pale or mottled color
    g. Mental confusion, syncope, dizziness
    h. Diaphoresis

Signs and Symptoms of Cardiac, Pulmonary and Venous Congestion
    a. Auscultation of an S_3 or S_4 gallop or both
    b. Orthopnea
    c. Rapid, often labored respirations
    d. Auscultation of rales
    e. Cough
    f. Peripheral edema, especially of dependent areas
    g. Increased jugular vein distention
    h. Hepatomegaly
    i. Anorexia

Signs and Symptoms of Pulmonary Edema
    a. Productive cough, frothy or blood-tinged sputum
    b. Summation gallop
    c. Nocturia, oliguria

Diagnostic Tests

Chest X-ray. This is routinely ordered for documentation of cardiomegaly, venous congestion of the pulmonary beds and pleural and pericardial effusions.

Electrocardiogram (ECG) and Cardiac Enzymes. These studies rule out the possibility of myocardial infarction.

Electrolytes.   Electrolytes, especially sodium and potassium, are indicators of degree of water excess. Serum potassium may be low if the patient has been on diuretics and replacement therapy has not been instituted.

Digoxin Level.   This study should be performed if the patient has been taking digitalis and there is evidence to suspect toxicity.

Hemodynamic Monitoring.   This provides an early and accurate means of estimating ventricular function. The following data demonstrate the use of the pulmonary artery wedge pressure (PAWP) as a guideline in assessing the progression of CHF.

PAWP	0 to 6 mm Hg	Reduction of circulating volume
PAWP	6 to 12 mm Hg	Within normal limit
PAWP	18 to 20 mm Hg	Onset of pulmonary congestion
PAWP	20 to 25 mm Hg	Moderate pulmonary congestion
PAWP	25 to 30 mm Hg	Severe pulmonary congestion
PAWP	>30 mm Hg	Pulmonary edema

COMPLICATIONS

Complications can be categorized as those resulting from the pathophysiology of CHF and those occurring secondary to treatment.

CHF-Induced Complications

Decreased Ability to Manage Activities of Daily Living.   A decline in abilities develops as cardiac reserve falls.

Arrhythmias.   These may occur in response to increased catecholamine release and myocardial ischemia. Prolonged atrial ischemia often leads to atrial fibrillation.

Angina and Myocardial Infarction.   These conditions result from an increased workload on an ischemic heart or from decreased coronary artery perfusion due to falling systemic pressure or from both.

Shock. This occurs as cardiac output drops.

Renal Failure. This condition follows a prolonged lack of adequate blood flow to the kidney.

Emboli Formation. This may result from venous stasis and congestion.

Treatment-Induced Complications

Hypovolemia. This may occur from overly vigorous diuretic therapy with excessive sodium and water loss.

Hypokalemia. This condition is a consequence of excessive potassium loss with diuresis through use of furosemide (Lasix), ethacrynic acid and thiazides, and it may potentiate arrhythmia.

Digoxin Toxicity. Toxicity may result from overmedication with digoxin, hypokalemia or failing renal function.

Arrhythmias. These may result from digoxin toxicity, diuretic-induced electrolyte imbalances and sympathomimetic agents.

Emboli Formation. This is enhanced when excessive diuretic therapy produces a higher hematocrit and greater blood viscosity. Bed rest, with increased venous stasis, also potentiates risk.

Myocardial Infarction. MI can occur as myocardial workload is increased by inotropic agents.

MEDICAL AND NURSING MANAGEMENT

The aim in the treatment of CHF is to decrease demands on the left ventricle and increase its O_2 supply. This may be accomplished by decreasing preload, decreasing afterload and increasing contractility. As noted earlier, these three factors are interrelated and are the primary determinants of the amount of blood that will be ejected with each heartbeat. As always, the precipitating causes should be identified and concurrently treated.

Decreased Preload

1. In an emergent situation, circulating volume may be rapidly decreased by the use of phlebotomy.

2. More frequently, however, potent intravenous diuretics such as furosemide (Lasix), 20 to 80 mg, as needed, are used to decrease the venous return. It should be noted that if a profound diuresis is accomplished by phlebotomy, it may precipitate circulatory collapse. Furosemide is also used at times with aminophylline for a cumulative effect and to increase diuresis.

3. Body position may also decrease venous return. A high Fowler's position decreases the amount of circulating volume returning to the heart and also causes the diaphragm and abdominal contents to drop, allowing for better aeration. The preferred position is often one in which the patient leans forward with the arms and head on an overbed table padded with pillows.

4. Rotating tourniquets are an immediate method of decreasing venous return. Tourniquets or blood pressure (BP) cuffs may be used. They are placed high on three or four extremities, and every 5 to 15 minutes one is tied while another is untied in either a clockwise or a counterclockwise rotation. An arterial pulse should be palpable on the tied extremity. If BP cuffs are used, the pressure should be set at the patient's diastolic level. As the clinical situation improves, the tourniquets are released one at a time.

5. The use of intravenous morphine (3 to 10 mg) also creates venous pooling. It has additional benefits: It relieves pain (which results from ischemia) and reduces anxiety, causing a decrease in outpouring of catecholamines.

6. A direct effect of the use of nitroprusside-dopamine therapy is a decrease in preload. The nitroprusside (Nipride) causes an increase in venous capacitance, whereas small doses of dopamine (Intropin) cause renal vasodilation and thus increase renal blood flow, the glomerular filtration rate and sodium excretion.

7. Recently, nitroglycerin, especially in IV form (50 mcg q 3 to 5 min or 5 to 20 mcg per min IV drip via infusion pump), has been used effectively to decrease the preload in patients with CHF or pulmonary edema associated with acute MI.

Decreased Afterload

Afterload can be decreased by the use of agents, such as morphine, nitroglycerin, which reduces arteriolar resistance, or Laxis, which reduces circulating volume.

Increased Contractility

1. Myocardial contractility may be increased by the use of intravenous digitalis (digoxin) (digitalizing dose to total 0.5 to 2 mg; maintenance dose, 0.125 to 0.5 mg qd). Not only will its positive inotropic effect increase pump efficiency, but its vagal effect on decreasing heart rate (especially in atrial fibrillation) will also allow for better perfusion of the coronary arteries by increasing the length of diastole.

2. Intravenous aminophylline (250 mg in 100 to 200 ml D_5W IV drip) is sometimes utilized for its beta effect on increasing contractility, dilating the bronchioles (if wheezing occurs) and increasing renal blood flow. However, its positive effects may be outweighed by the negative, in that it may concurrently increase heart rate and myocardial irritability, thus increasing O_2 demand on an already failing heart.

3. Since ischemia may impair the heart's ability to contract, the use of oxygen is imperative. This may range from the use of nasal oxygen via prongs to endotracheal intubation and a ventilator. Arterial blood gases (ABG) and the clinical situation may be used as a guide to determine the route and amount of oxygen needed.

Supportive Measures

1. Rest is of primary importance because it decreases myocardial oxygen demands and the stimulus for aldosterone production that is triggered by standing.

2. The issue of psychological support in dealing with a patient who is experiencing CHF cannot be overemphasized. The feeling of "not being able to get one's breath" is terrifying, and to the patient, death seems imminent. This patient needs constant reassurance that he or she is, in fact, not dying. The sedative effect of morphine may be most beneficial in this instance. It is also important to explain all procedures to the patient and the

benefits of each in a simple, concise manner. Stress and fear cause an increased release of catecholamines and aldosterone, further taxing the failing heart.

3. Vital signs should be checked frequently, as they are indicative of progress or deterioration in the patient's condition.

4. Hemodynamic monitoring may be well utilized to dictate the direction of therapy. PAWP reflects preload status, and cardiac output (CO) reflects the actual efficiency of the pump.

5. Daily weights or intake and output, or both, should be monitored to aid in understanding the patient's fluid status. A baseline weight should be obtained on admission if possible.

6. A low-sodium diet or fluid restriction or both may be indicated to aid in maintaining appropriate circulatory volume and electrolyte balance.

7. Cardiac monitoring should be utilized, as shifts in clinical lab values and medication side effects may cause arrhythmia.

8. The need for use of energy-conserving measures in dealing with these patients is obvious. All activities should be considered and adequately spaced to allow for maximum utilization of oxygen by the myocardium with a minimal amount of effort.

9. Electrolytes should be monitored closely during diuresis, as potassium stores may deplete rapidly, leaving the patient increasingly susceptible to digitalis toxicity.

10. Temporary use of anticoagulants (heparin, 5000 units q 8 hours SC) is sometimes advocated. The CHF patient is more susceptible to venous thrombosis because of increased venous congestion. Excessive clotting also may result from overly vigorous diuresis.

11. Teaching the patient in regard to long-term maintenance of the therapeutic program should be stressed in order to prevent rehospitalization.

SUGGESTED READINGS

Braunwald, E.: *Heart Disease*. Philadelphia, W. B. Saunders, 1980.

Dracup, A.: Physiologic basis for combined nitroprusside-dopamine therapy in post myocardial infarction heart failure. *Heart and Lung*, 10:114, 1981.

Forrester, J. S., et al.: Hemodynamic therapy of myocardial infarction. *N. Engl. J. Med.*, 295:1356, 1976.

Foster, S. B., and Canty, K.: Pump failure following myocardial infarction: an overview. *Heart and Lung*, 9:293, 1980.

Malin, C.: New concepts in understanding congestive heart failure. Part 1: How clinical features arise. *Am. J. Nurs.*, 81:119, 1981.

Malin, C.: New concepts in understanding congestive heart failure. Part 2: How therapeutic approaches work. *Am. J. Nurs.*, 81:357, 1981.

14

SHOCK

GENERAL CONSIDERATIONS

Definition

Shock is a clinical syndrome caused by a discrepancy between the vasocapacity and the circulating volume, resulting in redistribution of body fluid and hypoperfusion of tissue. Few acute physiological conditions so profoundly affect as many vital body systems as does shock.

Classification

There are four major categories according to etiology: cardiogenic, hypovolemic, septic and neurogenic. Although cardiogenic shock is most often encountered in coronary care settings, it is important to be able to differentiate between the types of shock. This chapter, therefore, will present all shock syndromes while focusing on cardiogenic shock.

ETIOLOGY

The etiologies of shock syndromes are significantly different. Specific causes of shock are listed in Table 14–1.

Cardiogenic Shock

Cardiogenic shock is caused by severe pump failure. Myocardial infarction with loss of more than 40 per cent of the left ventricular muscle mass is the most common cause.

Hypovolemic Shock

Hypovolemic shock is caused by loss of 15 to 20 per cent of intravascular volume, either internally or externally.

Septic Shock

Septic shock is caused by bacterial endotoxins that result in massive vasodilation and increased venous capacitance.

Neurogenic Shock

Neurogenic shock is caused by sudden loss of vasomotor tone throughout the body, leading to increased venous capacitance as a result of depression of or damage to vasomotor centers.

PATHOPHYSIOLOGY

Pathogenesis

Cardiogenic Shock.   Cardiogenic shock begins with a significant decrease in cardiac output caused by pump failure. This leads to diminished circulating volume, decreased blood pressure (BP) and increased peripheral vascular resistance (PVR), resulting in tissue hypoperfusion.

Hypovolemic Shock.   Hypovolemic shock begins with diminished circulating volume caused by loss of blood or intravascular volume. This leads to decreased BP and increased PVR, resulting in tissue hypoperfusion.

Septic Shock.   The development of septic shock is quite different. It begins with vasodilation and normal or increased cardiac output and blood pressure. The body's response to endotoxins causes vasodilation, lowering peripheral vascular resistance, and damages capillary endothelial cells, increasing permeability. The leakage of intracapillary plasma to the interstitial spaces leads to circulatory collapse, resulting in *hypoperfusion* as seen in cardiogenic and hypovolemic shock.

Neurogenic Shock.   Neurogenic shock begins with decreased PVR from sudden loss of vasomotor tone. This leads to peripheral pooling, which decreases venous return. The resultant fall in cardiac output causes tissue hypoperfusion.

Pathophysiological Consequences

Regardless of etiology, the major pathophysiological consequences of shock syndrome are due to hypoperfusion. The body responds to hypoperfusion via a series of compensatory mechanisms.

Compensatory Mechanisms
Activation of the Sympathetic Nervous System.   This is due

Table 14–1. CAUSE AND TREATMENT OF SHOCK

TYPE	CAUSE	TREATMENT
Cardiogenic*	Pericardial tamponade	Volume (crystalloids, colloids)
	Massive pulmonary embolism	Catecholamines (vasopressors)
	Valvular obstruction—clot	Nitroprusside (Nipride)/furosemide (Lasix)
	Rapid tachycardias	Glucocorticoids
	Arrhythmias	Oxygenation
	Myocardial infarction with 40 per cent of myocardium	IABP
	Rupture of chordae tendineae	Surgery
	Papillary muscle dysfunction	Treat precipitating cause
	Acute myocarditis	
	Terminal heart failure	
Hypovolemic*	Hemorrhage—gastrointestinal (GI) bleeding or trauma	Trendelenburg position
	Plasma loss—burns	Volume (crystalloids, colloids, blood products)
	Dehydration—diabetes mellitus, heat exhaustion, vomiting, diarrhea, Addison's disease	Vasopressors
		Glucocorticoids
		Oxygenation
		Antishock (MAST) trousers
		Treat the cause:
		Stasis of bleeding
		Reduction of GI loss
		Autotransfusion

| Septic† | Gram-negative bacteremia (*Escherichia coli, Klebsiella, Pseudomonas, Proteus, Serratia*) Gram-positive bacteremia (*Streptococcus, Staphylococcus*) Yeast, fungal infection | Volume (crystalloids, colloids) Antibiotics Beta-agonists Oxygenation Positive end-expiratory pressure (PEEP) for adult respiratory distress syndrome (ARDS) Platelets for disseminated intravascular coagulation (DIC) Glucocorticoids Antishock trousers Vasopressors |
| Neurogenic† | Brain stem injury, spinal anesthesia or spinal cord injury, deep anesthesia, pain, drugs, heat stroke and insulin shock | Treat the cause: Relief of pain Reverse narcotic effect Airway management Antishock trousers Vasopressors Oxygenation Volume (crystalloids, colloids) |

*Shock with decreased circulating volume.
†Shock with increased vasocapacity.

to hypotension, which triggers the baroreceptor reflex. This reflex results in peripheral arterial and venous constriction, increased heart rate and myocardial contractility.

Activation of Renin-Angiotensin-Aldosterone System.   This activation is due to renal ischemia, which causes the release of renin and in turn the production of angiotensin II. This causes further vasoconstriction and stimulates the release of aldosterone, which enhances sodium and water retention by the kidneys.

Stimulation of the Pituitary Gland.   This stimulation results in anterior pituitary release of adrenocorticotrophic hormone (ACTH), which stimulates increased release of aldosterone from the adrenal cortex. This, in turn, increases renal sodium and water retention. The posterior pituitary releases antidiuretic hormone (ADH), which increases water reabsorption by the kidney. This mechanism attempts to expand the circulating volume.

Redistribution of the Body Fluid.   Redistribution is accomplished by reabsorbing large amounts of intestinal and interstitial fluids into the intravascular beds in an attempt to expand the circulating volume.

Metabolic and Tissue Changes

If the compensatory mechanisms accounting for many of the signs and symptoms seen in shock are not interrupted by therapeutic means as early as possible, they will perpetuate, with uncontrollable pathological consequences.

Lactic Acidosis.   Ischemia enhances incomplete oxidation at the cellular level. Anaerobic metabolism of glucose leads to accumulation of lactic acid and profound metabolic acidosis. Vasodilation results from the release of vasoactive substances such as bradykinin, histamine, serotonin and prostaglandins.

Tissue and Organ Damage

Heart.   Increased cardiac workload, resulting from the compensatory increase in PVR, heart rate and myocardial contractility, may cause cardiac ischemia, rhythm disturbances and pump failure.

Kidneys.   Decreased renal perfusion leads to acute tubular necrosis (ATN) and renal failure. The appearance of oliguria (<30 ml/hour) is followed by anuria (<100 ml/24 hours).

Brain.   Decreased cerebral perfusion results in restlessness followed by apathy or stupor.

Intestine.   Splanchnic ischemia causes increased susceptibility for bacteria and toxins to cross the intestinal barrier and enter the circulation, leading to sepsis and vasodilation.

Liver. Impaired hepatic cells have a decreased ability to produce energy and detoxify circulating toxins. In addition, blood is sequestered in larger amounts in the liver. Ischemic hepatic cells also release lysosomes into the circulation, further damaging capillary walls.

Lungs. The release of vasoactive substances and proteolytic enzymes results in interstitial leakage and pulmonary congestion (adult respiratory distress syndrome).

Capillaries. Acidosis and circulatory toxins damage capillary endothelial cells. This facilitates plasma protein and fluid leakage into the interstitial spaces, resulting in interstitial edema and hypovolemia.

Platelets. Vasoconstriction and sluggish blood flow leads to platelet aggregation and microthrombi. Disseminated intravascular coagulopathy (DIC) may result.

Cells. Total cellular deterioration is caused by profound ischemia. Lysosomes, which are intracellular "stomachs," break down and release proteolytic enzymes. Active transport is impaired, and sodium with water accumulates in the cells, causing them to swell and die.

PATIENT ASSESSMENT

Intial assessment should include identifying the underlying event so that the cause and the consequence can be treated concurrently. Clinical evaluation and hemodynamic monitoring form the basis for diagnosis and management of the patient in shock. Comparative signs and symptoms of the various types of shock are listed in Table 14–2.

DIAGNOSTIC TESTS

Electrolytes. Assess fluid and electrolyte shifts.

Blood Counts. Rule out bleeding and sepsis.

Electrocardiogram (ECG) and Cardiac Enzymes. Rule out myocardial infarction.

Chest X-ray and Arterial Blood Gas (ABG). Monitor pulmonary ventilation and perfusion status.

Table 14–2. SIGNS AND SYMPTOMS OF SHOCK

SYSTEM CHANGES	CARDIOGENIC	HYPOVOLEMIC	SEPTIC	NEUROGENIC
Neurologic	Extreme fatigue Restlessness Apprehensiveness Drowsiness Stupor Coma	Same	Same	Same
Cardiovascular	Normal—low BP, ↓ pulse pressure (PP) (early) ↓ Cardiac output (CO) ↑ Peripheral vascular resistance (PVR) ↑ Pulmonary artery wedge pressure (PAWP) Rapid pulse—thready Slow capillary refill Distended jugular veins (later)	↓ BP ↓ PP (early) ↓ CO ↑ PVR ↓ PAWP Rapid, thready pulse Slow capillary refill Flat jugular veins	↓ BP ↓ PP (late) ↑ or ↓ CO ↓ PVR ↓ PAWP Rapid pulse Slow capillary refill Flat jugular veins	↓ BP ↓ PP (late) ↓ CO ↓ PVR ↓ PAWP Normal—slow pulse Slow capillary refill Flat neck veins

Respiratory	Tachypnea Rales	Tachypnea Clear (initially)	Tachypnea Clear (initially)	Varies with neurologic disorders Clear (initially)
Renal	*Early:* Oliguria (<30 ml/hour) *Late:* Anuria (<100 ml/24 hours)	Same	Same	Same
Skin	Cool, moist Cyanosis/pallor	Cool, moist Pallor Poor turgor	Dry, warm Flushed, pale Cyanosis (late) Poor turgor (late)	Dry, warm Pale, pink Cyanosis (late) Poor turgor (late)
Miscellaneous	Nausea ↓ Bowel tones ↓ or ↑ Temperature Metabolic acidosis (late)	Nausea Thirst, ↑ temperature ↓ Bowel tones Metabolic acidosis (late)	Nausea ↓ or ↑ Temperature ↓ Bowel tones Metabolic acidosis (late)	↓ Bowel tones ↓ or ↑ Temperature Metabolic acidosis (late)

Creatinine and Blood Urea Nitrogen (BUN). Evaluate renal function and rule out impairment.

Hemodynamic Monitoring. Provides information for differential diagnosis of shock states and aids in evaluating therapy. A cardiac index of less than 2 liters/minute/m^2 is indicative of shock.

COMPLICATIONS

Shock-Induced Complications

See discussion under Metabolic and Tissue Changes.

Treatment-Induced Complications

Complications of treatment should be assessed and weighed against clinical benefits.

Renal Failure. This may be potentiated through use of vasopressors (e.g., levarterenol bitartrate [Levophed] or high-dose dopamine) secondary to increased renal shunting.

Heart Failure and Pulmonary Edema. These can occur after overaggressive fluid resuscitation, especially in the compromised heart.

Coagulopathy. This disorder is a concern as calcium levels fall after massive transfusion of citrated blood (in hypovolemic shock).

Infection. This is always possible when invasive therapy is instituted, i.e., intravenous lines, hemodynamic monitoring, catheterization, intubation, and so on.

Local Tissue Necrosis and Sloughing. These can occur after infiltration of a potent vasoconstrictor such as levarterenol bitartrate (Levophed).

MEDICAL AND NURSING MANAGEMENT

The main focus of therapy in all types of shock is to treat the cause. However, in cardiogenic shock, since the primary cause is irreversible loss of adequate left ventricular function, the mortality rate remains 80 per cent.

Volume Regulation

Frank hypovolemia is rarely the cause of shock in a coronary patient, although it may occur secondary to overvigorous diuresis. Continuous monitoring of vital signs usually will reflect the presence of postural hypotension early in the course, and volume deficits may be dealt with before they become life threatening. If the pulmonary artery wedge pressure (PAWP) is low or below therapeutic limits (18 mm Hg), a fluid challenge may be tried to take full advantage of Starling's law. This is usually instituted in the form of dextran or normal saline in boluses of 100 to 200 ml over 10 minutes to an hour. Should the PAWP rise and remain 18 mm Hg and clinical signs of shock persist (in absence of pulmonary hypertension), volume replacement is not the answer. If the PAWP rises well above therapeutic levels, diuretics may be necessary to return to the therapeutic range.

Catecholamines

Catecholamine therapy is directed at maintaining an arterial pressure of 90 to 100 mm Hg to ensure adequate tissue perfusion. Dopamine, norepinephrine, and dobutamine are the commonly used agents.

1. Dopamine (Intropin) is administered intravenously as a continuous drip. With small doses, 3 to 10 mcg/kg/minute, an inotropic effect is achieved, increasing the arterial pressure while allowing for selective perfusion of the kidneys. The concurrent use of nitroprusside (0.5 to 8 mcg/kg/minute), which is a vasodilator, and dopamine may be initiated to decrease afterload as well as increase contractility. Careful titration and attention to the PAWP, as well as to the vital signs, are necessary to achieve the proper pharmacological balance. Diastolic blood pressure of 60 mm Hg should be maintained to ensure coronary artery perfusion.

2. Norepinephrine (Levophed) is administered by intravenous drip at 2 to 8 mcg/minute to achieve more of an alpha-adrenergic effect. Phenotolamine (Regitine) is used to prevent tissue necrosis in case of extravasation of norepinephrine into the tissue. Regitine is injected directly into the area of extravasation.

3. Dobutamine is administered by intravenous drip at 2.5 to 10 mcg/kg/minute. It primarily stimulates beta-adrenergic

inotropic receptors in the heart with minimal chronotropic or peripheral vasodilatory effects.

4. The use of isoproterenol (Isuprel) is contraindicated with the patient in cardiogenic shock unless an atropine-resistant bradycardia is present and pacing is not available.

Glucocorticoids

The use of glucocorticoids in cardiogenic shock is controversial. Their exact effect is not fully understood. Among the possible effects, a few are currently thought to be stabilizing of lysosomal membranes, preventing the release of histamine and bradykinin and preventing excessive lactate accumulation.

Digitalis

The use of digitalis is also subject to controversy. The positive inotropic effect has to be weighed against the increased myocardial oxygen demand it creates. Patients in shock are more prone to digitalis toxicity owing to potassium shifts.

Oxygenation

It is imperative to combat hypoxia, to maintain a PO_2 greater than 80 mm Hg. Supplementary oxygen may be delivered in the form of nasal prongs. Mechanical ventilation may be necessary, should respiratory failure occur.

pH Correction

Acidosis is corrected to reach and maintain a pH of 7.35. Intravenous sodium bicarbonate in boluses of 45 mEq is given intermittently to maintain a correct pH.

Mechanical Circulatory Assistance

In selected cases, intra-aortic balloon counterpulsation pump (IABP) is used to increase oxygen supply to the myocardium while reducing the heart's oxygen demand. It increases coronary artery blood flow during diastole and decreases afterload during systole, thus reducing myocardial oxygen consumption. See Chapter 21.

Surgery

Catastrophes such as intraventricular septum perforation, ruptured papillary muscle and dissecting aortic aneurysm all decrease the pumping efficiency of the heart and may require emergent surgical intervention. Coronary artery bypass graft may also be attempted in an effort to salvage ischemic yet viable left ventricular muscle. The ultimate surgical intervention is heart transplant.

Pericardial Tap

Pericardial tap is indicated if the cause of shock is cardiac tamponade.

Arrhythmia

Cardioversion or use of antiarrhythmic drugs or both are recommended for life-threatening tachycardias, whereas pacing is the treatment of choice for life-threatening bradycardias or for overriding a tachycardia.

Nutrition

The patient in shock should be kept NPO to rest the hypoperfused bowel. The use of hyperalimentation should be used to aid in the prevention of a catabolic state.

Psychological Support

The patient experiencing cardiogenic shock may be hurting, confused, withdrawn and appropriately afraid that he is dying. Morphine, given intravenously in small doses, will help to alleviate pain and anxiety as well as cause vasodilation and a decrease in the outpouring of catecholamines. The nurse should maintain a calm, supportive attitude; touch alone may be an important factor. The nurse should explain all procedures and therapies in concise, simply understood terms to the patient and significant others, as their level of anxiety may interfere with their comprehension. The nurse should also encourage the patient and the family to verbalize their fears and feelings.

Aggressiveness of Treatment

Although current therapies are available, they remain very costly. Therefore, the appropriateness of treatment must be carefully weighed early in the course. Important factors to be considered include the patient's age, the general state of health prior to admission and the prognosis for quality of life. The final decision regarding aggressiveness of treatment should be the result of open discussion between the nurse, physician, patient and patient's significant others. The role of the nurse is a central one because he or she must coordinate communication between the involved parties while providing support during this difficult time.

SUGGESTED READINGS

Crumlish, C. M.: Cardiogenic shock—catch it early! *Nursing '81*, 11:34, 1981.

De Sanctis, R. W.: Shock. In *Scientific American Medicine*, Section I, Vol. I, *Cardiovascular Medicine*. New York, Scientific American, 1981.

De Wood, M. A., et al.: Intra-aortic balloon counterpulsation with and without reperfusion for myocardial infarction shock. *Circulation*, 61:1105, 1980.

Dracup, K. A., Breu, C. S., and Tillish, J. H.: The physiologic basis for combined nitroprusside-dopamine therapy in post myocardial infarction heart failure. *Heart and Lung*, 10:114, 1981.

Forrester, J. S., et al.: Hemodynamic therapy of myocardial infarction. *N. Engl. J. Med.*, 295:1356, 1976.

Guyton, A.: *Textbook of Medical Physiology*, 6th ed. Philadelphia, W. B. Saunders, 1981, pp. 332–343.

Schumer, W.: Septic shock. J.A.M.A., 242:1906, 1979.

Sumner, S. M., and Grau, P. A.: To defeat hypovolemic shock—anticipate and act swiftly. *Nursing '81*, 11:47, 1981.

15

HYPERTENSION

GENERAL CONSIDERATIONS

Definition

According to the Joint National Committee on Detection, Education and Treatment of High Blood Pressure, hypertension is defined as systolic/diastolic pressure of 160/95 mm Hg or more. The American Heart Association further defines high blood pressure as 140/90 mm Hg in individuals under 20 years of age.

Significance

Hypertension is the most significant risk factor for heart failure, renal failure and stroke. These disorders constitute the leading causes of death in the United States. Hypertension causes great reduction in life expectancy if left untreated; the higher the pressure, the worse the prognosis.

Classification

Hypertension is classified according to etiology and severity.

According to Etiology

Primary (Essential or Idiopathic) Hypertension. The cause is unknown. It encompasses 90 to 95 per cent of the hypertensive population.

Secondary Hypertension. The cause is identifiable. It encompasses 5 to 10 per cent of the population. Etiologies are listed in Table 15–1.

According to Severity

Malignant (Accelerated, Acute) Hypertension. Blood pressure accelerates to 200/140 mm Hg or above. It occurs as a clinical crisis, threatening severe damage to organs and organ systems. Death will follow unless immediate aggressive therapy is instituted.

Borderline (Labile) Hypertension. This may be mild or intermittent, the blood pressure fluctuating between normal and abnormal. Typically, diastolic readings are between 90 and 95 mm Hg. Patients in this group should be considered

Table 15–1.   CAUSES OF SECONDARY HYPERTENSION

I. *Systolic and Diastolic Hypertension*
  1. *Renal hypertension*
      Parenchymal diseases:
        Chronic pyelonephritis
        Congenital renal diseease
        Diabetic nephropathy
        Glomerulonephritis
        Polycystic kidney
        Renin-secreting tumor
      Vascular hypertension
  2. *Endocrine hypertension*
      Cushing's syndrome
      Primary hyperaldosteronism
        Conn's syndrome
        Idiopathic hyperaldosteronism
      Pheochromocytoma
  3. *Coarctation of the aorta*
  4. *Drug-induced hypertension*
      Oral contraceptives
      Estrogens, steroids
      Thyroid hormones
      Amphetamines
  5. *Pregnancy-induced hypertension*
  6. *Neurogenic*
      Psychogenic
      Increased intracranial pressure
  7. *Miscellaneous*
      Increased intravascular volume
        Polycythemia vera
        Postoperative
      Burns
      Carcinoid syndrome
II. *Systolic Hypertension*
  1. *Increased cardiac output*
      Aortic regurgitation
      Arteriovenous fistula
      Patent ductus arteriosus
      Thyrotoxicosis
      Paget's disease of bone
      Beriberi
      Hyperkinetic circulation
      Anemia
  2. *Rigidity of the aorta*

for an early and effective control program in order to curtail the potential for adverse progressions.

ETIOLOGY

Primary Hypertension

Although the cause is unknown, primary hypertension is strongly associated with various factors such as positive family history, salt intake, obesity, occupation, age, race, sex, smoking, serum cholesterol level and diabetes mellitus.

Secondary Hypertension

The elevation of blood pressure is secondary to an existing disorder, as listed in Table 15–1.

PATHOPHYSIOLOGY

Implicating Factors

The pathophysiology of hypertension is not fully understood; however, it can be traced to disorders in the normal mechanisms of blood pressure control. Blood pressure equals cardiac output times total peripheral resistance ($BP = CO \times TPR$) and is further affected by blood volume and viscosity. The following factors are implicated in creating an imbalance of the BP equation.

1. Normal cardiac output and increased peripheral resistance.
2. Increased cardiac output and normal peripheral resistance.
3. Elevated plasma renins.
4. Increased angiotensin II.
5. Elevated mineralocorticoids (aldosterone).
6. Retention of salt and water by the kidneys, which normally excrete salt and water when blood pressure rises.
7. Salt sensitivity combined with an excessive salt intake.
8. Increased basal sympathetic activity.
9. Pathological responses to stress with outpouring of catecholamines.
10. Lack of vasodilator substances (prostaglandins, kinins).
11. Combined volume excess and vasoconstriction.

Pathological Changes

Sustained hypertension eventually leads to pathological changes. The medial layer of the arteries is the most affected, undergoing edema and then hypertrophy. The increased pressure on the arteries causes microaneurysms and small hemorrhages. The atherosclerotic process is accelerated. Plaque formation and sclerosis of arterial vessels lead to narrowing and tortuosity, resulting in ischemia to the areas supplied.

PATIENT ASSESSMENT

Owing to the insidious and silent nature of the disease, the patient usually appears asymptomatic. Careful assessment of a hypertensive patient is necessary and should include history, physical assessment and laboratory studies.

Patient History

The history should include the following data:

1. Previous documentation of high blood pressure, including prescribed medical regimen.
2. Family history of hypertension, diabetes and cardiovascular disease.
3. History of any disease or trauma to target organs.
4. Presence of cardiovascular disease.
5. Symptoms of cardiovascular disease.
6. Ingestion of substances associated with hypertension, such as birth control pills, estrogens, steroids, thyroid hormone, diet pills, cold capsules, amphetamines, cocaine and large amounts of licorice.
7. Description of lifestyle, including occupation, diet, sodium intake, leisure activities and stress level.

Physical Assessment

Physical assessment should include proper determination of blood pressure as well as evaluation of target organs.

Taking Blood Pressure. Using the proper techniques described in Chapter 1, blood pressure should be taken at least twice on each arm, on three separate occasions, to confirm the diagnosis of hypertension (BP $\geq$ 160/95 mm Hg). If a high reading is obtained once, suspect labile hypertension.

Once hypertension is diagnosed, trends in blood pressure should be identified by taking serial blood pressures at regular intervals over a 24-hour period. This procedure is recommended for patients on antihypertensive medications to identify peaks and troughs that may require adjustment in therapy.

Assessment of Target Organs. Sustained hypertension involves pathological changes that affect target organs and organ systems. Therefore, the organ systems should be evaluated separately. Pathological signs and symptoms may be noted as follows in the target organs (See Table 15–2).

COMPLICATIONS

High blood pressure is a primary contributor to at least one third of premature cardiac deaths and an even larger percentage of cerebral vascular deaths.

Hypertension-Induced Complications

Complications of hypertension tend to occur late in the disease process and are seen in the following target organs:

Heart
Coronary Artery Disease (CAD). Development of this disease is enhanced threefold.
Angina Pectoris and Myocardial Infarction. These may occur as coronary artery blood flow decreases.
Left Ventricular Failure. This often follows increased afterload with increased myocardial oxygen demands.
Arrhythmia and Sudden Death. These can result from all the preceding reasons.

Brain
Strokes. These can occur by two mechanisms:
Multiple Microaneurysms. These result in intracerebral hemorrhage.
Transient Ischemic Attacks or Cerebral Infarction. These may occur in the wake of advanced atherosclerosis.
Hypertensive Encephalopathy. This is associated with a temporary rise in arterial pressure, leading to confusion, convulsions and coma.

Kidney
Renal failure may occur secondary to progressive nephrosclerosis and focal necrosis of renal arterioles.

Table 15–2. PHYSICAL ASSESSMENT AND DIAGNOSTIC PROCEDURES OF TARGET ORGANS

TARGET ORGAN	PHYSICAL ASSESSMENT	POSSIBLE DIAGNOSTIC PROCEDURES
Brain	Headache: throbbing and occipital on awakening (fades after patient is up awhile) Changes in mentation (speech, memory, temperament) Sensory and motor deficits (gait, coordination) Convulsions Coma	Spinal tap Computerized tomographic (CT) scan
Eyes	Visual disturbances (blurring, dim spots) Blindness Changes in ocular fundi—ranging from minimal narrowing of retinal arteries in relation to veins (Grade I) to papilledema with extensive hemorrhage and exudate (Grade IV)	
Heart	Chest pain S_3 gallop and rales (congestive heart failure, or CHF) Dyspnea S_4 gallop (atrial enlargement) Palpitations Enlarged point of maximal impulse (PMI) Peripheral edema	Chest X-ray (heart size, lung congestion) ECG: Amplitude of QRS (left ventricular hypertrophy, or LVH) prolonged, m-shaped or biphasic P waves (atrial enlargement) Arrhythmias

Vessels	Acute chest pain or abdominal pain (dissecting aneurysm) Weak peripheral pulse Bruits Intermittent claudication Hemorrhage Discoloration of the skin	Cholesterol Triglycerides Chest X-ray (size and shape of great vessels)
Kidneys	Palpably enlarged kidney Nocturia Fatigue or weakness Peripheral edema	Electrolytes: Na^+, K^+ (hyperaldosteronism) Creatinine, blood urea nitrogen (BUN), uric acid level PRA (stimulated plasma renin activity) Urinalysis: hematuria, proteinuria, sedimentation, intravenous pyelography (IVP)
General Considerations		Complete blood count (CBC) (anemia, polycythemia) Fasting blood sugar (FBS) (diabetes, Cushing's syndrome) Calcium (hyperparathyroidism) Urine: VMA (vanillylmandelic acid) metanephrines (pheochromocytoma)

Others

Intermittent Claudication.   This occurs when atherosclerosis involves the aorta and arteries of the lower extremities.
Dissecting Aortic Aneurysm.   This results from hypertensive damage to the aortic wall.

Treatment-Induced Complications

A variety of complications can result from treatment of both chronic and acute hypertension. They usually occur as exaggerated side effects from antihypertensive drugs.

Hypokalemia.   This is the most common complication associated with diuretic therapy.

Vertigo and Syncope.   These conditions are indicative of postural hypotension and can be seen with use of diuretics, methyldopa, guanethidine, trimethaphan and prazosin.

Sexual Dysfunction.   Sexual dysfunction in the form of decreased libido and impotence is a side effect of most sympathetic agents and vasodilators. Guanethidine can also cause retrograde ejaculation.

Gastrointestinal Disturbances.   Gastrointestinal disturbances such as nausea, vomiting and diarrhea are commonly seen with most antihypertensive drugs. Paralytic ileus is of concern with guanethidine use. Peptic ulcer is a common side effect of reserpine.

Depression and Sleep Disturbance.   Depression and sleep disturbance (i.e., nightmares) are seen with sympathetic agents, especially reserpine.

Reflex Tachycardia and Palpitations.   These are major occurrences with the use of vasodilator agents: prazosin, hydralazine, minoxidil, diazoxide and nitroprusside.

Weight Gain.   Weight gain from fluid retention is an adverse effect on the beta-blockers, guanethidine and other sympathetic agents.

Fatigue and Drowsiness.   These increase the safety risk and can occur as blood pressure falls with any antihypertensive agent (methyldopa and clonidine more than others).

Dry Mouth and Frequent Voiding. These are effects of diuretic therapy.

Headache. Headache, often frontal or global, is a side effect of vasodilation agents.

Fasting Hypoglycemia. Can occur with beta blockers.

MEDICAL AND NURSING MANAGEMENT

A major problem in the treatment of hypertension is an unwillingness on the part of patients to comply with treatment regimens. Many treatment methods impact directly on the patient's lifestyle, in areas difficult to change. These include dietary restriction (sodium and calorie), smoking and stress reduction. Many antihypertensive medications have unsavory side effects, which, when combined with the fact that hypertension itself often has no annoying symptoms, makes it very tempting to disregard treatment programs. Hypertension is easily ignored until it produces pathological conditions or complications that change the perceived severity of the disease. Compliance is highly dependent on the patient's understanding and perception of hypertension and its consequences; this makes education of the patient an important part of the treatment program. The treatment program should include specific goals of maintaining blood pressure within a given range. Nonpharmacological methods are the first choice. If the goal cannot be maintained, then pharmacological methods are used.

Nonpharmacological Methods of Treatment

Weight Control. A significant decrease in mean blood pressure can be accomplished with a weight loss of 15 to 30 pounds without undergoing any sodium restriction. Although weight loss alone is not recommended for treatment, it is certainly indicated as part of a treatment program.

Dietary Sodium Restriction. Lowering the dietary intake of sodium from 3500 to 5000 mg per day to 1000 to 2000 mg per day may lower the blood pressure as much as 10 mm Hg. Treatment includes recognition and avoidance of foods high in sodium. Physicians may order 24-hour urine samples to measure sodium content in a diet.

Alcohol and Coffee Restriction.   Moderate alcohol use need not be prohibited. It is recommended that not over 2 oz a day be consumed; heavier drinking increases the likelihood of hypertension. Caffeine raises the blood pressure by activation of the sympathetic nervous system and should be avoided.

Exercise.   Isometric exercising should be avoided, as blood pressure rises during isometric contraction. Consistent exercise programs that involve aerobic exercising for a minimum of 1 hour three times a week have been shown to lower blood pressure.

Smoking.   The physiological effects of smoking include an increased heart rate and peripheral vasoconstriction, both of which contribute to elevated blood pressure.

Stress Reduction and Relaxation Techniques.   Stress reduction may be aimed at identifying and modifying stressful factors in a person's lifestyle and at scheduling of time for more leisure activities. "Type A" personalities have a higher incidence of hypertensive disease. Therapy with these patients may be directed at their emotional status. Relaxation techniques have been found to be a useful tool in the control of mild-to-moderate hypertension. Biofeedback techniques can be taught to patients in short periods of time.

Patient Teaching.   It is crucial that the patient fully understand the consequences of uncontrolled hypertension and the body's response to prescribed medications. The patient should also be instructed to self-monitor the blood pressure. This includes taking the blood pressure, keeping an accurate daily record, and recognizing and documenting situations that precipitate elevation in blood pressure. Teaching of the patient should also include any necessary modifications of lifestyle.

Pharmacological Methods of Treatment

Control of hypertension is frequently dependent on pharmacological agents—namely, diuretics, sympatholytics and vasodilators. These agents work by decreasing blood volume, cardiac output or peripheral resistance. Diuretics reduce circulatory volume. Sympatholytics lower peripheral resistance and cardiac output. Vasodilators work directly to decrease peripheral resistance. The pharmacological agents are

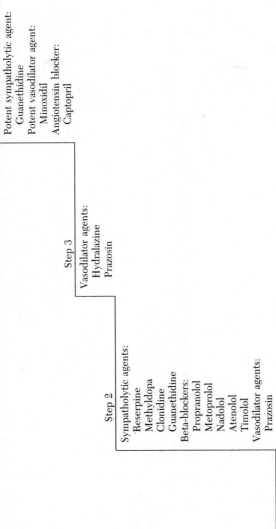

Figure 15–1. The step care approach to initiating nonemergent antihypertensive therapy.

Step 1

Diuretic agents
  (plus potassium replacement):
Thiazides:
  Hydrochlorothiazide
  Chlorothiazide
  Chlorthalidone
Loop diuretic:
  Furosemide

Step 2

Sympatholytic agents:
  Reserpine
  Methyldopa
  Clonidine
  Guanethidine
Beta-blockers:
  Propranolol
  Metoprolol
  Nadolol
  Atenolol
  Timolol
Vasodilator agents:
  Prazosin

Step 3

Vasodilator agents:
  Hydralazine
  Prazosin

Step 4

Potent sympatholytic agent:
  Guanethidine
Potent vasodilator agent:
  Minoxidil
Angiotensin blocker:
  Captopril

Table 15–3. DRUGS FOR TREATMENT OF HYPERTENSIVE EMERGENCY

| MEDICATION | METHOD OF ADMINISTRATION | | ONSET OF ACTION | SIDE EFFECTS |
	Dose, IM	Dose, IV		
Direct vasodilators				
Hydralazine (Apresoline)	10–60 mg	Intermittent, 20–40 mg/20 ml (1 ml/minute);	IM, 30 minutes IV, 10 minutes	Tachycardia, angina, lupus-like symptoms
Diazoxide (Hyperstat)	—	Intermittent, 300 mg rapidly	1–5 minutes	Hyperglycemia, GI distress, sodium retention, tachycardia
Sodium nitroprusside (Nipride)	—	Continuous, 50–150 mg/liter, (3 mcg/kg/m)	Instantly	Signs of cyanide poisoning, severe hypotension, angina, tachycardia, acute tubular necrosis

Sympathetic agents				
Reserpine (Serpasil)	1–5 mg	—	2–3 hours	Somnolence, mental depression, nightmares
Ganglionic blocking agents				
Trimethaphan (Arfonad)	—	Continuous, 1000 mg/liter (3–4 mg/min), titrate	5–10 minutes	Postural hypotension, paralytic ileus, visual disturbances
Methyldopa (Aldomet)	—	Intermittent, 250–500 mg/100 ml (over 30–60 minutes)	4–6 hours	Impotence, postural hypotension, hemolytic anemia, depression
Phentolamine (Regitine)	5–20 mg	Intermittent, 2–5 mg (rapidly)	IV, instantly IM, 5 minutes	Arrhythmias and acute prolonged hypotension
Loop Diuretics				
Furosemide (Lasix)	—	Intermittent, 40–80 mg	5 minutes	Hypovolemia, hypokalemia, hyperglycemia, hyponatremia, hypochloremia, alkalosis
Ethacrynic acid (Edecrin)	—	Intermittent, 50 mg	5 minutes	

used in both maintenance control and hypertensive emergencies.

Maintenance Control. Patients who are on maintenance control of hypertension can be on any one drug or a combination of antihypertensive medications. When a patient is initially diagnosed as having hypertension, a drug therapy program must be chosen. The goal of therapy is effective control of blood pressure with a minimum of side effects. The Step Care Approach, as recommended by the Joint National Committee on Detection and Control of Hypertension, is usually used. (See Fig. 15–1.) The patient is started on Step 1, which is a diuretic, usually a thiazide. The drug is gradually increased to a maximum dosage. If blood pressure is not controlled, a Step 2 agent may be used or added to the Step 1 drug. Higher step (Steps 3 and 4) medications are tried until control is achieved. Choices of medications are based on the type of hypertension (systolic, diastolic or both), the age of onset, severity and coexisting conditions that would contraindicate certain medications. Interactions with other drugs the patient may be taking should also be considered.

Hypertensive Emergency. The goal of treatment of the patient in hypertensive crisis is immediately to reduce the blood pressure enough to remove the threat of death or catastrophic effect on target organs. Treatment is dependent totally on parenteral administration of medications (See Table 15–3). Most often, two or three agents are used concurrently. A diuretic should always be used in conjunction with an antihypertensive agent.

Treatment of Secondary Hypertension

The management of secondary hypertension is directed at treating the cause. Medications that are specific to the causative organ systems are used. When appropriate, surgical intervention is indicated. Otherwise, palliative therapy, similar to that used in primary hypertension, is the only feasible approach.

SUGGESTED READINGS

Braunwald, E. (ed.): *Heart Disease*. Philadelphia, W. B. Saunders, 1980.
Grim, C. M.: Nursing assessment of patients with high blood pressure. *Nursing Clin. North Am.*, 16:349, 1981.

Haber, E., and Slater, E. E.: High blood pressure. *Scientific American Medicine*, Section I, Vol. I, *Cardiovascular Medicine*. New York, Scientific American, 1981.

Hartshorn, J. C.: What to do when the patient is in hypertensive crisis. *Nursing '80*, 10:36, 1980.

Hutchins, L. N.: Drug treatment of high blood pressure. *Nursing Clin. North Am.*, 16:365, 1981.

Kochar, M. S., and Daniels, L. M.: *Hypertension Control*. St. Louis, C. V. Mosby, 1978.

Marcinek, M. B.: Hypertension—what it does to the body. *Am. J. Nurs.*, 80:925, 1980.

Phillips, R.: *Cardiovascular Therapy: A Systemic Approach*. Philadelphia, W. B. Saunders, 1979.

The 1980 Report of the Joint National Committee on Detection, Evaluation and Treatment of High Blood Pressure. National Heart, Lung and Blood Pressure Institute, National High Blood Pressure Education Program. Bethesda, Md., Institutes of Health, 1980, 20205.

16

MISCELLANEOUS DISORDERS

The miscellaneous disorders included in this chapter may occur as an acute coronary event secondary to myocardial infarction or concurrently with myocardial infarction, or as a chronic condition requiring lifelong adaptation. Detailed nursing assessment aids in diagnosis and proper management of these less frequently encountered cardiac disorders.

Pericarditis and Cardiac Tamponade

PERICARDITIS

DEFINITION

Pericarditis is inflammation of the sac surrounding the heart, the pericardium.

ETIOLOGY AND INCIDENCE

Pericarditis can be caused by bacterial or viral infections, myocardial infarction, neoplastic disease and trauma or may occur after cardiac surgery.

Infectious Pericarditis

Infectious pericarditis results when pathogenic organisms invade the pericardium. The Coxsackie group B viruses are the most common pathogens. It has been calculated that up to one third of patients infected with these viruses develop symptoms of pericarditis. Mycotic and rickettsial infections are rarely implicated.

Post–Myocardial Infarction Pericarditis

This type of pericarditis is seen as an early complication of acute myocardial infarction. The incidence has been reported to be between 7 and 16 per cent of all patients with myocardial infarction (MI). Autopsy reports indicate that a large number of pericarditis cases are missed. Pericarditis after MI most frequently occurs after acute anterior transmural infarcts, rarely with subendocardial infarcts, and is due to epicardial leakage of blood into the pericardium.

Dressler's Syndrome

Dressler's syndrome, or post–myocardial infarction syndrome (PMIS), differs from acute pericarditis in that the etiology is thought to be from a late-appearing autoimmune response to myocardial necrosis. The symptoms usually appear 3 to 6 weeks after MI and last much longer than symptoms of acute pericarditis. The incidence of Dressler's syndrome is 1 to 4 per cent of all MI patients.

Neoplastic Pericarditis

Neoplastic pericarditis is due to invasion of the pericardium by malignant tumors of adjoining structures.

Hemorrhagic Pericarditis

Hemorrhagic pericarditis may ensue after trauma to the chest that causes blood to escape into the pericardial sac.

Metabolic Pericarditis

Metabolic pericarditis can follow uremia and myxedema.

PATHOPHYSIOLOGY

The pericardium is composed of two layers, an inner serous membrane (epicardium) and a fibrous sac (parietal pericardium). The space between these two layers is the pericardial cavity, which normally contains 15 to 50 ml of clear, serum-like fluid that serves as a lubricant. When the pericardial cells are injured, they release a combination of fluid, fibrin and cells in an inflammatory response. The serofibrous exudate roughens the two layers and creates friction between them. There is often irritation and inflammation of the surrounding pleura and diaphragmatic tissues.

PATIENT ASSESSMENT

Physical Findings

Pain. Pericardial pain typically is located in the anterior precordium and radiates to the shoulders, although it may occur in many other locations. It is usually aggravated by deep breathing, swallowing and coughing and is sometimes relieved by leaning forward. The character is variable, from a deep, dull, constant ache to sharp or burning pain. It often is not relieved by nitroglycerin or morphine. Pain usually appears 4 to 48 hours before a rub is heard.

Friction Rub. In most cases, pericarditis is diagnosed by the appearance of the rub, usually appearing on the second or third day after MI. The sound of the rub can be scratching, grating, crunching or squeaking and is best heard at the left mid to lower sternal border, with the patient leaning forward or lying in the left lateral position to bring the heart in contact with the anterior chest wall. The rub may have varying components. A three-component rub reflects the heart's movement during atrial systole, ventricular systole and ventricular diastole. Two-and-one component rubs may be difficult to distinguish from murmurs. The quality and intensity is variable, explaining why they disappear and reappear. They do not vary with respiration, nor do they radiate.

Fever. The body temperature is usually less than 39°C (102°F).

Dyspnea and Tachypnea. These can be secondary to avoiding the pain of deep breathing.

Restlessness, Irritability and Anxiety. These traits may develop owing to the reappearance of distressing chest pain and stimulation of the sympathetic nervous system.

Diagnostic Tests

Electrocardiogram (ECG). See Fig. 16–1. There is a concave ST segment elevation on limb and precordial leads.

Chest X-ray. This is used to rule out cardiac tamponade.

Complete Blood Count (CBC). A CBC may reveal elevated WBC count.

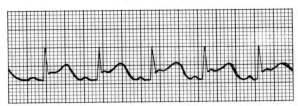

Figure 16–1. Concave upward ST segment elevation in pericarditis.

Erythrocyte Sedimentation Rate (ESR). This value is usually elevated.

Serologic Viral Studies. These studies are used to rule out Coxsackie virus. They require serum from the acute and convalescent stages taken 2 weeks apart.

Chemistry Profile. This is used to identify metabolic causes.

COMPLICATIONS

Arrhythmias

Arrhythmias may be due to irritation of the sinus node, which is located close to the parietal pericardium. Atrial arrhythmias, especially atrial flutter, and atrioventricular (AV) conduction disturbances result.

Cardiac Tamponade (see below.)

MEDICAL AND NURSING MANAGEMENT

The treatment of pericarditis is symptomatic and oriented toward alleviating the pain and preventing complications.

Narcotics

Narcotics are given to control pain, although pericardial pain often will not respond to narcotics.

Anti-Inflammatory Agents

Anti-inflammatory agents are used to reduce the pain and inflammation. Indomethacin (Indocin), 50 mg t.i.d., is used first. Aspirin, 2 tablets q.i.d., may be used when pericardial bleeding is not suspected. If the pain is not relieved, steroids are used. Corticosteroid therapy can bring dramatic relief of pain within 30 minutes, although their use is controversial

owing to the side effects of hypertension and sodium retention.

Antibiotics

Antibiotics are used to treat infectious pericarditis.

Bed Rest

Bed rest is indicated during the acute phase.

Stress Reduction

Stress reduction is essential for the anxious patient in pain.

CARDIAC TAMPONADE

DEFINITION

Cardiac tamponade is fluid accumulation in the pericardium
of sufficient quantity to cause cardiac compression and prevent
normal diastolic filling of the heart.

ETIOLOGY

Cardiac tamponade can be caused by infection, neoplasm,
or trauma. It can also develop as a complication of pericarditis,
cardiac surgery, anticoagulation therapy or aortic dissection.

PATHOPHYSIOLOGY

Constriction of the heart within the pericardium results in
decreased cardiac output and eventually elevated systemic
venous pressure. The hemodynamic manifestations depend
on how rapidly the fluid accumulates. A rapid accumulation
of 100 milliliters can result in symptomatology, whereas slowly
developing tamponades have resulted in accommodation of
up to 2000 ml by the pericardial sac.

PATIENT ASSESSMENT

Clinical Presentations

Elevated Neck Veins.   This is due to congestion of the right
side of the heart and venous system.

Narrowed Pulse Pressure.   This is secondary to decreased cardiac output.

Pulsus Paradoxus.   A paradox of greater than 10 mm Hg is often present. (See Chapter 1.)

Distant or Inaudible Heart Sounds.   This is a common finding on auscultation.

Dyspnea.   Dyspnea is a result of decreased cardiac output and pulmonary congestion.

Cyanosis.   Cyanosis may be present if tissue perfusion is decreased.

Diagnostic Tests

ECG.   ECG demonstrate electrical alternans or low voltage.

Chest X-Ray.   An enlarged cardiac silhouette may be noted.

Echocardiogram.   This often provides the definitive diagnosis and an estimation of the amount of fluid in the pericardial sac.

MEDICAL AND NURSING MANAGEMENT

Bed Rest.   Bed rest, with head slightly elevated, is indicated. Milder tamponade may resolve with this conservative treatment.

Close Monitoring.   Close monitoring of the electrocardiogram and the vital signs is important to forewarn of worsening condition.

Pericardiocentesis.   Withdrawal of fluid from the pericardial sac is indicated in serious cases that present with life-threatening symptoms.

Surgery.   Creation of a pericardial window and continuous drainage of pericardial fluid into the intrapleural space may be indicated in recurrent tamponade.

_____ **Myocarditis** _____

DEFINITION

Myocarditis is defined as inflammation of the cardiac muscular tissue, the myocardium. Myocarditis can be acute or chronic.

ETIOLOGY AND INCIDENCE

Infectious Myocarditis

The cause of infectious myocarditis can be viral, bacterial, rickettsial, fungal, protozoal or metazoal. In North America, Coxsackie B virus is the most frequent cause of viral myocarditis. The myocardial membrane is particularly susceptible to viral particles. Myocarditis usually appears after a lag of several weeks after the initial infection, often following an upper respiratory infection or influenza. One third of fatal influenza cases show evidence of active myocarditis.

Noninfectious Myocarditis

Noninfectious myocarditis can be caused by factors in any of four categories.

Toxic, Chemical or Drug Effects. Myocarditis may be caused by phenothiazines, lithium carbonate, catecholamines and carbon monoxide.

Hypersensitivity Reactions. Reactions to methyldopa, penicillin, sulfonamides, tetracycline and other agents may produce myocarditis.

Physical Agents. Heat stroke, hyperthermia, hypothermia and radiation may result in myocarditis.

Metabolic Disorders. Myocarditis may be caused by lupus erythematosus, nephritis, uremia and diabetes.

PATHOPHYSIOLOGY

Myocarditis is an inflammatory process that may involve the myocytes, interstitium or vasculature. Infectious agents produce the damage by direct invasion, production of toxins or initiation of an autoimmune response. The myocardial involvement can be focal or diffuse. Necrosis can occur. Lesions are usually randomly distributed in the myocardium. The heart may remain normal in less serious cases, and in more severe ones it may dilate, hypertrophy or become flabby.

PATIENT ASSESSMENT

The symptoms depend on the location and size of the lesion. Myocardial involvement is subclinical in most cases, and patients offer no specific complaints. Diagnosis is then inferred from the changes on the electrocardiogram.

Physical Findings

Physical findings include dyspnea, palpitations and precordial discomfort due to inflammation. Patients with acute myocarditis present with cyanosis, weak peripheral pulses and low blood pressure. Chest pain often results from associated pericarditis. Tachycardia and elevated temperature are present. The first heart sound is often muffled, and a transient apical systolic murmur may appear.

ECG Changes

The ECG changes most commonly seen are nonspecific abnormalities of the ST segment and T wave. Q waves may appear. Ventricular arrhythmias are more common than atrial ones. If the lesion is in the conduction system, heart block may occur. AV conduction disturbances are common.

CBC

The WBC may be elevated.

Cardiac Enzymes

Cardiac enzyme levels are elevated, although not as much as with MI.

ESR

The ESR is moderately elevated for 2 to 3 weeks.

Ultrasound

Ultrasound may be used to evaluate the thickness of the myocardial wall and possible exudate accumulation in the pericardial sac.

COMPLICATIONS

Most patients recover completely.

Chronic Myocarditis.   Chronic myocarditis can develop after an acute episode.

Chronic Congestive Cardiomyopathy.   Chronic congestive cardiomyopathy can result from acute myocarditis.

Arrhythmias.   Arrhythmias, especially ventricular ones, can occur.

Complete AV Block.   Complete AV block is usually transient but can result in death.

Congestive Heart Failure.   Congestive heart failure occurs only in the severe cases.

Death.   Death results in 5 per cent of the cases of the viral form but can occur in any of the other forms.

MEDICAL AND NURSING MANAGEMENT

Treatment is supportive and is directed at the symptoms and accompanying condition, if any.

Absolute Bed Rest.   Absolute bed rest is essential, as it hastens recovery and reduces long-term damage to the myocardium.

Oxygenation.   Oxygenation is necessary if hypoxia is present, since hypoxia intensifies the damage.

Antiarrhythmics.   Antiarrhythmics are used for specific arrhythmias, although propranolol is avoided.

Corticosteroids.   Use of corticosteroids is controversial.

Antiviral Agents or Antibiotics.   These agents are used to treat infectious myocarditis.

Digitalis. Digitalis can produce toxicity easily in myocarditis, so it should be used with caution.

Diet. A light diet should be ordered.

Stress. Stress, both physical and emotional, should be reduced.

———— Infective Endocarditis ————

GENERAL CONSIDERATIONS

Definition

Infective endocarditis is defined as infection of the endocardium; the infection may be septal, mural or valvular, involving right, left or both sides of the heart.

Classification

1. Acute: may result in rapid, severe destruction of valve tissue.
2. Subacute: produces damage more slowly.

Incidence

Infective endocarditis is rare in children and is more common in men than in women. The age range is 31 to 60.

Predisposing Factors

1. Underlying heart disease—rheumatic valvular or congenital defects.
2. Prosthetic cardiac valve.
3. Intravenous (IV) drug addiction.

ETIOLOGY

Infective endocarditis results from transient bacteremia or fungemia, the causative organisms including staphylococcus, streptococcus, enterococcus, *Pseudomonas*, gonococcus and *Candida*. The same organism can cause acute or subacute endocarditis. The severity of the course taken by the disease depends on the patient's defense state as well as on the virulence of the organism.

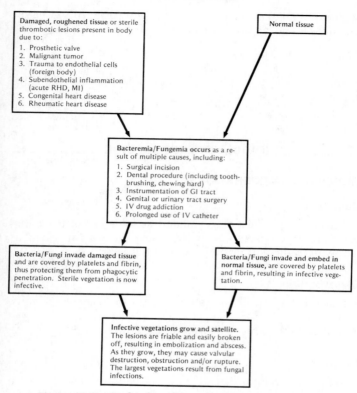

Figure 16–2. Pathophysiology of infective endocarditis.

PATHOPHYSIOLOGY

The pathophysiology of infective endocarditis involves the development of characteristic infective vegetations on valve leaflets or elsewhere in the endocardium. See Figure 16–2.

PATIENT ASSESSMENT

Signs and Symptoms

Infective endocarditis should be suspected in any patient who presents with a murmur and fever of unknown origin for 1 week. See Table 16–1.

Table 16–1. SIGNS AND SYMPTOMS OF INFECTIVE ENDOCARDITIS

	ACUTE ENDOCARDITIS	SUBACUTE ENDOCARDITIS
Onset	Abrupt	Gradual
Presentation	Acutely ill	Complaining of flulike symptoms (malaise, anorexia, fatigue, weight loss, aching muscles)
Fever (may not be present in patients with renal failure or CHF)	High temperature and chills common	Usually low-grade fever, remittent at night
Murmur (often regurgitant—may be absent in tricuspid involvement)	New or changing. If too acute, may not have had time to develop	Subtle, may not be present
Other	Any may be present	Any may be present
1. Splenomegaly		
2. Petechiae		
3. Splinter hemorrhages (dark red lines under fingernails and toenails)		
4. Roth's spots (retinal hemorrhages)		
5. Osler's nodes (painful intracutaneous papillae on pads of fingers and toes)		
6. Janeway's lesions (hemorrhages on palms of hands and soles of feet)		

Laboratory Data

Blood Cultures. At least two blood cultures should be done. They should demonstrate bacteremia or fungemia. The samples should be drawn multiple times before antibiotic therapy is initiated. If an acute process is suspected, obtain approximately six samples over a 2-hour period. If a subacute process is suspected, obtain approximately six samples over 2 to 3 days.

CBC. The CBC demonstrates normocytic, normochromic anemia. The WBC may be normal. The differential may be normal or may show a shift to the left.

Sedimentation Rate. This rate is almost always elevated.

Blood Urea Nitrogen (BUN) and Creatinine. These values are elevated in patients with severe renal complications.

Urinalysis. Urinalysis demonstrates proteinuria and hematuria.

Rheumatoid Factor. This factor is often positive in a subacute process.

Cerebrospinal Fluid (CSF). The fluid may show pleocytosis and protein.

Echocardiography

The echocardiogram suggests the location of vegetations 2 mm or larger.

COMPLICATIONS

Complications Due to Infective Endocarditis

1. Embolic episodes to vital organs, resulting in hemiplegia, blindness, flank pain or pleuritic pain.
2. Mycotic aneurysms, often in the brain, may rupture years later.
3. Abscesses anywhere in the body.
4. Myocarditis.
5. Myocardial infarction.
6. Valvular destruction, obstruction or rupture—drug addicts

usually complicate with tricuspid destruction, resulting in right endocarditis and pulmonary emboli.
7. CHF due to valvular involvement.
8. Renal failure.
9. Death, if untreated.

Complications Due to Treatment of Infective Endocarditis

These complications result from prolonged antibiotic therapy.

1. Rash.
2. Fever.
3. Hemolytic anemia.
4. Neutropenia.
5. Renal toxicity.
6. Ototoxicity.
7. Seizure activity.
8. Superinfection (from colonization of penicillin-resistant bacteria or fungi).

MEDICAL AND NURSING MANAGEMENT

Parenteral Antibacterial or Antifungal Therapy

This therapy is administered for 4 to 6 weeks, the agent or agents being specific to the sensitivity shown by the infective organism cultured. The usual initial regimen (pending identification of the organism) is IV penicillin, ± 2 million units every 4 to 6 hours, plus IV gentamicin, ± 80 mg every 8 hours, or penicillin as stated plus IV streptomycin, 0.5 to 1.0 gm every 12 hours. Vancomycin is used if the patient is allergic to penicillin. After the first 2 weeks, antibiotic therapy may be changed to the oral route. Effective drug management requires penetration of the infective vegetation in sufficient concentration to kill the bacteria or fungi. If the patient is an IV drug addict, or if there is an identified source of staphylococcus, methicillin, 2 gm IV every 4 hours, should be substituted for penicillin.

Anticoagulant

Use of anticoagulants is controversial owing to the increased risk of hemorrhage (especially intracranial).

Table 16–2. PROPHYLACTIC ANTIMICROBIAL REGIMENS TO PREVENT ENDOCARDITIS

PROCEDURE	ORGANISM	REGIMENS
Dental or ear, nose and throat procedures	S. viridans, microaerophilic streptococci, S. pneumoniae	Procaine penicillin G, 1.2 million units (300,000–600,000 units in children) IM given 30 to 60 minutes before the procedure. For major procedures, this dose should be repeated q 8–12 hours for 24 to 48 hours after the procedure. For minor procedures, or after procaine penicillin G is discontinued in major procedures, phenoxymethyl penicillin, 500 mg orally q.i.d. (125 to 250 mg orally q.i.d. in children), should be given until bleeding stops or the area is healing well.
	As above plus relatively resistant streptococci	In patients who are receiving regular parenteral benzathine or oral penicillins as prophylaxis against rheumatic fever: procaine penicillin G, 1.2 million units IM, plus methicillin, 1.0 gm IM. 30 to 60 minutes before the procedure. For a major procedure requiring hospitalization, aqueous penicillin G, 1 million units IV, plus methicillin, 1.0 gm IV, can be given just prior to the procedure and q 4 hours for 24 to 48 hours postoperatively. Oral treatment following the parenteral therapy in this situation should be cloxacillin, 500 mg orally q.i.d. (125 to 250 mg orally q.i.d. in children).

Patients allergic to penicillins can receive cefazolin,* 1.0 gm IM, instead of procaine penicillin, and erythromycin or cephalexin orally instead of phenoxymethyl penicillin or cloxacillin. Patients allergic to penicillins and cephalosporins should receive vancomycin,* 1.0 gm IV q 8 hours (250 to 500 mg IV q 8 hours in children), as the parenteral agent and erythromycin, 500 mg t.i.d. orally (125 to 250 mg t.i.d. orally in children).

Gastrointestinal, biliary and genitourinary procedures — Enterococcus (γ Streptococcus)

Ampicillin, 1.0 gm IM or IV, or amoxicillin, 0.5 to 1.0 gm (125 to 250 mg in children) orally 30 to 60 minutes before the procedure and amoxicillin in the same dosage t.i.d. orally until the bleeding has stopped or the manipulated area is healing well.

In high-risk (prosthetic valve) situations or with extensive manipulations, add gentamicin,* 60 to 80 mg IM 30 minutes before the procedure and q 8 hours for 24 to 48 hours.

IV ampicillin can be continued postoperatively if the patient is to be NPO for a period of time.

In patients allergic to penicillins, use vancomycin plus gentamicin prior to and following the procedure in the dosages given in paragraphs 3 and 4 above.

*See manufacturer's official directive for dosage in patients with impaired renal function. From Williams, T. W.: Infective endocarditis. In Conn, H. F. (ed.): Current Therapy 1982. Philadelphia, W. B. Saunders, 1982.

Surgical Intervention

Surgery may be necessary if a medical regimen fails, replacement of a prosthetic valve is needed or acute, severe valvular insufficiency occurs, necessitating implantation of a prosthetic valve. Fungal endocarditis almost always necessitates surgical intervention, often in the form of embolectomy to the extremities.

Close Observation

Close observation of vital signs and frequent physical assessment for appearance of or change in murmur, development of CHF and embolization.

Cardiac Monitor

Cardiac monitoring should be instituted to watch for appearance of intraventricular conduction defects or heart block due to septal abscess.

Teaching of the Patient

Teaching should stress the following:

1. Understandable explanation of the disease process and treatment.
2. Importance of prolonged antibiotic regimen to achieve sterilization of infective vegetations.
3. Importance of future prophylactic antibiotic therapy when undergoing dental manipulation or any surgical procedure or instrumentation. See Table 16–2 for recommended regimens.
4. Importance of routine clinical follow-ups after hospitalization for up to 6 months.

———— Rheumatic Heart Disease ————

GENERAL CONSIDERATIONS

Definition

Rheumatic heart disease is a chronic condition resulting from a delayed (months to years) sequela of rheumatic fever causing scarring and deformity of the heart valves.

Incidence

Rheumatic heart disease is considered to be the most frequent cardiac disorder in individuals under 40 years of age and second only to coronary and hypertensive heart disease in populations above 40 years of age. The most commonly affected valves are the mitral and aortic valves, especially in the combined form. Tricuspid involvement is less frequent and always coexists with mitral or aortic disorders. The pulmonic valve is rarely affected.

ETIOLOGY

Rheumatic Heart Disease

This disease is caused by rheumatic fever.

Rheumatic Fever

Rheumatic fever usually follows a beta-hemolytic group A streptococcal pharyngitis in a susceptible host (2 per cent of all people with "strep" throat). Rheumatic fever is an inflammatory disease process affecting various parts of the body,* with endocarditis being the most serious of all. Endocarditis causes valvulitis and eventually leads to permanent damage to the valves.

PATHOPHYSIOLOGY

Endocarditis (Valvulitis)

During this stage, the valvular cusps or leaflets and chordae tendineae are swollen and deposited with vegetations (bead-like) of platelets and fibrin, especially along the lines of valvular closure, leading to valvular and cardiac dysfunction.

Valvular Dysfunction

Scars formed after the acute valvulitis produce two types of dysfunction:

Stenosis.   The diffusely thickened fibrosis and calcified valve leaflets (cusps) gradually reduce the size of the orifice. The

---

*Other clinical features of rheumatic fever are polyarthritis, erythema marginatum, subcutaneous nodules and chorea. Minor features are fever, arthralgia, elevated ESR and prolonged P-R interval.

narrowed opening interferes with forward blood flow and leads to backward pressure buildup and various consequences, depending on the location of the valve.

Mitral Stenosis.   This gradually causes an increase of left atrial pressure. As the volume accumulates, the chamber becomes dilated and pulmonary congestion and eventually right heart failure will follow. Cardiac output may also decrease when the stenosis and the increased left atrial pressure fail to maintain left ventricular filling pressure.

Aortic Stenosis.   This causes increase of left ventricular pressure, which leads to increased myocardial workload and hypertrophy of the ventricular wall. When the oxygen demand exceeds the oxygen supply, myocardial ischemia and angina result. When the distensibility of the left ventricle decreases, cardiac output will also decrease, leading to hypoperfusion or syncope or both.

Tricuspid Stenosis.   This causes increase of right atrial pressure and leads to systemic venous congestion.

Regurgitation (Insufficiency).   The rigid and retracted leaflets (cusps) and the shortened chordae tendineae prevent the valve from closing properly. Therefore, blood flows backward from the high- to the low-pressure chamber. It leads to a series of consequences on either or both sides of the insufficiency.

Mitral Regurgitation.   This causes a greater dilatation of the left atrium than does mitral stenosis. The increased capacity permits a small pressure elevation in the left atrium and thus prevents significant pressure increase in the pulmonary capillary bed. The left ventricle also becomes dilated and hypertrophied owing to constant volume overload (normal plus regurgitant volume). Both mechanisms may maintain cardiac output at rest for a long time until heart failure eventually occurs. Then the pressures in the left atrium and pulmonary vasculature will increase and lead to right heart failure, as in mitral stenosis.

Aortic Regurgitation.   This permits blood to flow backward during systole and leads to left ventricular dilatation and then hypertrophy. When both mechanisms fail to maintain stroke volume, left heart failure results.

Tricuspid Regurgitation.   This allows volume and pressure increase in the right atrium, which leads to systemic venous congestion.

PATIENT ASSESSMENT

History-Taking

The history should include any incidence of childhood rheumatic fever, awareness of heart murmur, development of symptoms and the adaptation to the appearing symptoms.

Clinical Features

Patients with rheumatic heart disease are usually asymptomatic for many years. The appearance of symptoms usually occurs when the heart can no longer compensate for the increased pressure and workload (in or after the fourth decade). The characteristics of clinical presentation are dependent on the location of the valve and its nature of dysfunction. They are summarized in Table 16–3.

Diagnostic Tests

The findings of the commonly used tests are also summarized in Table 16–3.

COMPLICATIONS

Rheumatic Heart Disease–Induced Complications

Arrhythmias
Atrial Fibrillation. Atrial fibrillation is a common finding, especially in mitral valve disorders. It is believed to be caused by overstretching of the atrium. Atrial fibrillation with rapid ventricular rate often precipitates pulmonary edema because it reduces the ventricular filling time.

Ventricular Arrhythmias. These may be present in aortic disorders and may pose a threat to life.

Embolism. This is caused by dislodged thrombi from the fibrillating atrium (more often) or the calcified valve. It may lead to cerebral and myocardial infarction.

Congestive Heart Failure
Left Heart Failure. This occurs commonly in mitral regurgitation, aortic stenosis and regurgitation when the left ventricle begins to decompensate. It may eventually lead to right heart failure.

Right Heart Failure. This occurs commonly in mitral stenosis as a result of pulmonary hypertension and congestion.

Table 16–3. CLINICAL MANIFESTATIONS AND DIAGNOSTIC TESTS OF RHEUMATIC HEART DISEASE

AREAS OF ASSESSMENT	MITRAL STENOSIS (MS)	MITRAL REGURGITATION (MR)	AORTIC STENOSIS (AS)	AORTIC REGURGITATION (AR)	TRICUSPID STENOSIS (TS)	TRICUSPID REGURGITATION (TR)
Symptoms and observable signs	1. Signs of LVH: exertion, dyspnea, fatigue, coughing, orthopnea, paroxysmal nocturnal dyspnea (PND), hemoptysis 2. Palpitation—irregular pulse 3. Malar flush 4. Low normal BP 5. Signs of RVF may be present	1. Same as in MS except its progression is slower and milder	1. Onset of symptoms heralds increased risk of sudden death 2. Angina, syncope 3. Signs of LVH 4. Low pulse pressure	1. Could be asymptomatic despite poor LV function 2. Signs of LVF 3. Syncope and angina—rare 4. Wide pulse pressure 5. Waterhammer pulse (initially brisk→fades away suddenly)	1. Signs of systemic venous congestion: neck vein distention with giant "a" wave, hepatomegaly, RUQ pain, anorexia, ascites, peripheral edema 2. Often associated with MS	1. Same as in TS with signs of systemic venous congestion
Heart sound	1. Loud S_1 2. Opening snap after S_2 3. Low-pitched diastolic murmur at apex 4. Holosystolic murmur of TR	1. Soft S_1 2. Holosystolic murmur at apex—radiating to axilla 3. S_3 and S_4	1. Normal S_1 2. ↓ or absent aortic component of S_2 3. Rasping, crescendo-decrescendo systolic murmur—right sternal border radiating to neck 4. S_3 and S_4	1. Soft S_1 2. Loud S_2 3. High-pitched diastolic murmur—left lower sternal border 4. S_3 and S_4	1. Rumbling diastolic murmur—left sternal border, increases with inspiration	1. Holosystolic murmur—LLSB, increases with inspiration
Precordial impulse	1. Small or absent apical impulse 2. Palpable right ventricular impulse	1. Hyperdynamic apical impulse (↑ LV) 2. Para-sternal impulse (↑ LA)	1. Enlarged, sustained apical impulse 2. Systolic thrill right in second intercostal space	1. Large and diffuse diastolic thrill—left sternal border	1. Same as in MS if it coexists with MS	1. Palpable right ventricular impulse

ECG	1. P mitrale—enlarged left atrium 2. RVH pattern 3. Atrial fibrillation	1. P mitrale 2. LVH pattern 3. Atrial fibrillation	1. P mitrale 2. LVH pattern 3. LBBB/RBBB 4. AV conduction delay	1. LVH pattern	1. Tall, peaked P wave—right atrial enlargement	1. Tall, peaked P wave 2. RVH pattern
Chest X-ray	1. Left atrial enlargement 2. Pulmonary venous hypertension 3. May be enlargement of right atrium and ventricle	1. Left atrial and ventricular enlargement 2. Pulmonary vascular engorgement	1. Calcification of aortic valve 2. Left ventricular enlargement 3. Prominent ascending aorta	1. Left ventricular enlargement 2. Calcification of aortic valve 3. Dilatation of ascending aorta	1. Right atrial enlargement	1. Enlargement of right atrium and ventricle
Echocardiogram	1. Severity of stenosis 2. Size of left atrium 3. Right ventricular enlargement	1. Size of left atrium and ventricle 2. Bizarre motion of the leaflets	1. Fibrotic and calcified aortic valve 2. Severity and size of stenosis	1. Dilated and hyperdynamic left ventricle 2. Enlargement of aortic root and left atrium 3. Early closure of mitral valve	1. Motion and thickened tricuspid valve	1. Right ventricular dilatation 2. Paradoxical septal motion 3. Valvular thickening and motion
Cardiac catheterization	1. ↑ Left atrial pressure 2. Pressure gradient across mitral valve 3. Size of orifice 4. Pulmonary vascular resistance	1. Amount of regurgitant flow 2. Rule out prolapse and congenital disorders	1. Pressure gradient across aortic valve 2. Size of orifice	1. ↑ Left ventricular end-diastolic pressure 2. ↓ Aortic diastolic pressure 3. Amount of regurgitant flow 4. Left ventricular function	1. Pressure gradient across tricuspid valve	1. ↑ Right atrial pressure

Right heart failure (RHF) is the main complication of tricuspid regurgitation.

Infective Endocarditis. This occurs readily in patients with rheumatic heart disease when proper prophylactic measures are not employed.

Syncope. Syncope is experienced more often by patients with aortic stenosis than by those with aortic regurgitation. It is usually caused by

   a. AV block or atrial or ventricular arrhythmias.
   b. Restricted cardiac output insufficient for sudden increased activity level.

Angina. This is often experienced by patients with aortic stenosis when the restricted cardiac output fails to meet the myocardial oxygen demand.

Hemolytic Anemia. This is caused by the breakdown of red blood cells resulting from the turbulence around the deformed valve.

Treatment-Induced Complications

Hypovolemia and Hypokalemia. Either or both may occur owing to excessive diuresis.

Surgery-Induced Complications
Hemolytic Anemia. This can also be caused by the replaced prosthetic valve.
Infection on the Prosthesis. This infection often resists the previously used antibiotics and requires valve replacement again.
Clotting and Thrombosis at the Base of the Prosthetic Valve. Clotting and thrombosis may lead to valve malfunction and systemic embolism.
Parabasilar Leaks. These may occur around the suture line. Reoperation for repairment may be needed.

MEDICAL AND NURSING MANAGEMENT

Prevention of Recurrent Attacks of Rheumatic Fever and Infective Endocarditis

   1. Prophylactic antibiotics should be used with dental or surgical procedures (see Infective Endocarditis section of

this chapter). For instance, administer penicillin G (1 million units aqueous mixed with 600,000 units of procaine) IM, 30 minutes to 1 hour prior to the procedure, and then give penicillin V, 500 mg orally q 6 hours for eight doses.

2. Patient should be well taught and assisted to follow the prescribed medical regimen.

Activity

No limitation is necessary in asymptomatic individuals. Physical exertion, however, should be avoided in patients with moderate-to-severe aortic stenosis. All patients should be questioned carefully about their changing (if any) and current activity level. Marked limitation of activity is an indication for surgical therapy.

Diet and Fluid Management

Moderate restriction (no added salt) of sodium intake is indicated for patients with symptoms of pulmonary congestion. Fluid restriction, accurate intake/output documentation and daily weight measurements are essential for preventing, detecting and monitoring CHF.

Digitalis

Digitalis is used to control rapid ventricular response in atrial fibrillation and to maintain the heart rate at 60 to 80 beats per minute. It is also indicated when signs and symptoms of left ventricular failure are present. The usual daily dose of digoxin after digitalization is 0.125 to 0.25 mg PO.

Diuretics

Diuretics may be administered concomitantly with digitalis for patients with pulmonary congestion and peripheral edema. Careful observation is necessary for identifying signs of hypovolemia and decreased cardiac output (↑ fatigue) induced by overdiuresis. Furosemide (Lasix), 40 to 80 mg PO q d or b.i.d., is usually used. Daily potassium supplementation is often needed for patients receiving diuretics.

Vasodilators

Vasodilators may be added to lower the afterload in patients with refractory signs and symptoms of left ventricular failure despite the administration of digitalis and diuretics. A maintenance of systolic pressure at 90 to 100 mm Hg is used to regulate the dosage of the vasodilator. Isosorbide dinitrate, 5 to 10 mg SL q 4 to 6 hours or 20 to 40 mg PO q 6 hours, or hydralazine, 25 to 100 mg PO t.i.d., or both, may be selected.

Anticoagulants

Long-term oral warfarin may be used for patients with atrial fibrillation and a markedly enlarged atrium in order to prevent thrombi formation. Dosage is determined by prothrombin time. Patients should be taught to use guaiac for detecting blood in stools.

Antiarrhythmics

Sinus rhythm may sometimes be restored from atrial fibrillation by oral quinidine, 200 to 400 mg PO q 6 hours after digitalization. Ventricular ectopies and tachycardia are usually controlled by lidocaine, procainamide, disopyramide or quinidine as specified in Chapter 12.

Cardioversion

Cardioversion is often used to restore sinus rhythm before or after quinidine is tried for atrial fibrillation.

Surgery

Surgery is indicated when signs and symptoms of left ventricular decompensation appear. The decision for surgery in aortic valve disease (specially aortic stenosis) is much more urgent and definitive than that for mitral valve disease because rapid deterioration ensues once symptoms develop. The common surgical procedures are as follows:

Valvuloplasty.   This is performed only on selected patients with minimal or no valve calcification. It is usually done for patients with simple mitral stenosis. During this procedure, the adhesion of the mitral orifice is lysed mechanically.

Valve Replacement.   This is performed during open heart surgery for replacing the stenotic or regurgitant valve with a prosthetic plastic, metal or tissue valve. Lifetime anticoagulant therapy is usually continued for patients with mechanical valve replacement or persistent atrial fibrillation and enlarged atrium. The surgical mortality rate for valve replacement is 5 to 10 per cent.

Cardiomyopathy

DEFINITION

Cardiomyopathy refers to a large, miscellaneous group of degenerative myocardial diseases that interfere with the contractile function of the myocardium, resulting in pump failure.

CLASSIFICATION AND ETIOLOGY

On the basis of clinical and hemodynamic features, cardiomyopathy can be divided into three main categories:

Congestive Cardiomyopathy

The cause is generally unknown. In a minority of patients, causes may include beriberi (thiamine deficiency), thyrotoxicosis, various neuromuscular disorders, viral infections, diabetes mellitus, atherosclerotic heart disease, pregnancy and prolonged exposure to toxins such as alcohol or cobalt.

Restrictive Cardiomyopathy

Its cause is not clearly understood; however, it is associated with an infiltrative or fibrotic process within the myocardium. It is often confused with constrictive pericarditis. Causes may include amyloidosis, hemachromatosis, glycogen storage disease, sarcoidosis and neoplasm.

Hypertrophic Cardiomyopathy

Also called idiopathic hypertrophic subaortic stenosis (IHSS), hypertrophic cardiomyopathy is characterized by a disproportional hypertrophy of the ventricular septum resulting from an unknown cause. It is thought to have familial tendencies. Hypertrophic cardiomyopathy is discussed in the next section.

PATHOPHYSIOLOGY

Congestive heart failure is the common endpoint for all cardiomyopathies. It is the underlying pathologic process that differs among them. In congestive cardiomyopathy, there is significant fibrosis and hypertrophy of the myocardial fibers. This results in gross cardiomegaly (two to three times normal size) with a dilated and poorly contracting ventricle. Ventricular end-diastolic volume is high, and myocardial stretch exceeds the limits for a compensatory increase in force of contraction. Cardiac output falls below normal, and congestive heart failure ensues. In restrictive cardiomyopathy, the degree and type of fibrotic infiltration into the myocardium, endocardium and subendocardium cause the myocardium to lose its ability to stretch, thus impeding ventricular diastolic filling. Although contractility may remain normal, filling pressure increases and cardiac output falls. Eventually, hypertrophy and cardiac failure occur.

PATIENT ASSESSMENT

Physical Findings

Both congestive and restrictive cardiomyopathy show signs of cardiac biventricular failure: fatigue, dyspnea, orthopnea, pulmonary rales, pulsus alternans, jugular vein distention, ascites, hepatomegaly, peripheral edema, S_3 and S_4 gallops and high pulmonary artery wedge pressures (PAWP). These findings are usually more severe in congestive cardiomyopathy. Congestive cardiomyopathy may also precipitate nonspecific chest pain and prominent abnormal apical impulses (ventricular heaves). In both types of cardiomyopathy, murmurs of mitral and tricuspid regurgitation may be found. This is a result of dilation of the valvular anulus secondary to ventricular dilation.

Electrocardiography

Changes on ECG include low-voltage QRS complexes, nonspecific ST-T wave abnormalities, ventricular and atrial arrhythmias and conduction defects (usually left bundle branch block or degrees of AV block). Congestive cardiomyopathy may produce changes of left ventricular hypertrophy.

Echocardiography

This typically reveals left atrial enlargement and left ventricular dilation and hypertrophy with decreased contractile function. It helps in ruling out valvular disease and is the chief tool for diagnosing restrictive cardiomyopathy.

Angiography

Findings of enlarged heart cavities, poor contractions and generalized hypokinesia are consistent with congestive cardiomyopathy. These are absent in restrictive cardiomyopathy.

Isotope Scanning

The finding is characterized by generalized decrease in left ventricular contractility. Left ventricular formation is determined by calculating the ejection fraction.

COMPLICATIONS

Complications are the same as those for congestive heart failure (see Chapter 13). Ventricular arrhythmias may lead to lightheadedness, syncope or sudden death. Because of gross heart enlargement, mural thrombi are a constant threat to those with congestive cardiomyopathy. Even with intensive treatment, prognosis is poor. Postpartum cardiomyopathy is the exception, since patients may go into remission.

MEDICAL AND NURSING MANAGEMENT

Alleviation of Congestive Heart Failure

Alleviation of CHF is the usual aim of therapy. This is done with diuretics, digitalis and a low-sodium (less than 5 gm) diet.

Vasodilators

Vasodilators such as hydralazine (10 to 50 mg q.i.d. PO) prazosin (1 to 2 mg t.i.d. PO) and isosorbide dinitrate (5 to 60 mg q.i.d. PO) may be used for their beneficial effects in decreasing left ventricular preload and afterload. An added benefit is increased subendocardial perfusion. Nitroprusside

IV infusion (0.5 to 8 mcg/kg/minute) may be used in the acutely ill patient.

Treatment of the Cause

If a cause is known, treatment should be attempted—e.g., stopping alcohol ingestion or initiating anticancer therapy for neoplastic disorders.

Antiarrhythmic Drugs and Pacemaker Insertion

Antiarrhythmics and occasionally pacemaker insertion may be necessary as the rhythm disturbance dictates.

Anticoagulants

Anticoagulants are used to decrease the risk of thromboemboli.

Steroids

Steroids such as oral prednisone may be tried in patients with end-stage congestive cardiomyopathy in whom conventional methods are not working. Transient improvement may be seen.

Bed Rest

Bed rest and a marked decrease in physical activity are essential until clinical improvement occurs, as there is little cardiac reserve. This may take several months and is often not well tolerated emotionally.

Cardiac Transplantation

Cardiac transplantation can occasionally be offered to young individuals without other complicating medical conditions. It is, however, a costly procedure and carries a high risk of physical and emotional complications.

Teaching of the Patient

Teaching should stress avoidance of situations likely to precipitate failure, e.g., severe stress, discontinuance of medications, excessive sodium intake, alcohol abuse and pregnancy. Good nutrition should also be emphasized.

Idiopathic Hypertrophic Subaortic Stenosis (IHSS)

GENERAL CONSIDERATIONS

Definition

Idiopathic hypertrophic subaortic stenosis (IHSS) is a cardiomyopathy characterized by hypertrophy of the left ventricle, usually with disproportionate involvement of the intraventricular septum relative to the left ventricular free wall (see Fig. 16–3). It is also known as asymmetric septal hypertrophy (ASH), hypertrophic cardiomyopathy and hypertrophic obstructive cardiomyopathy (HOCM).

Significance

This cardiomyopathy carries with it the risk of sudden death, even though the patient may not be symptomatic.

ETIOLOGY AND INCIDENCE

In some, IHSS is inherited (non–sex-linked autosomal dominant). The basic causative defect is unknown. It often presents in young adults, the majority of cases being discovered in patients in their 30s and 40s; however, the age may range from birth to 85 years.

PATHOPHYSIOLOGY

The left ventricular hypertrophy results in displacement of the anterior leaflet of the mitral valve against the thickened septal wall during systole, causing a dynamic obstruction of the left ventricular outflow tract (Fig. 16–3). The degree of obstruction is dependent upon left ventricular volume, which is affected by preload, afterload and left ventricular contractility.

PATIENT ASSESSMENT

Symptoms

The most common presenting symptom is dyspnea. Other symptoms include angina, fatigue, palpitations, dizziness,

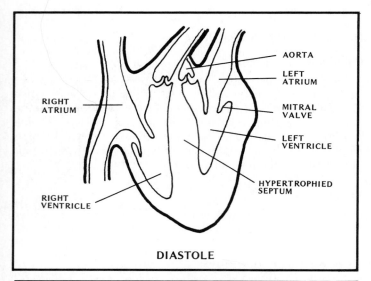

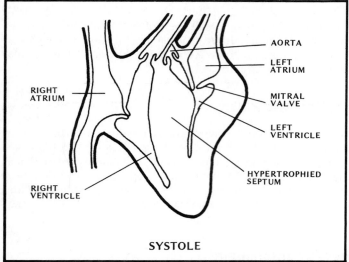

Figure 16–3. Hypertrophied intraventricular septum in IHSS.

"graying out" spells, syncope, paroxysmal nocturnal dyspnea and congestive heart failure.

Palpation and Visual Examination

PMI. The PMI is usually of increased force, enlarged and displaced laterally. A prominent presystolic apical impulse may be palpated. A systolic thrill is felt at the apex or left lower sternal border.

Left Ventricular Lift.   A left ventricular lift is often palpated.

Carotid and Peripheral Pulses.   These pulses usually demonstrate a brisk upstroke.

A Prominent "a" Wave.   A prominent "a" wave is often noted in the jugular pulse.

Auscultation of the Precordium

Loud S_4.   A loud S_4 is usually auscultated. S_3 may be present.

Systolic Murmur.   A systolic murmur of Grade 3 to 6 or greater is typically auscultated. It is harsh, crescendo-descrescendo and labile in intensity and duration. It is best auscultated at the apex and left sternal border, since it usually does not radiate into the neck.

ECG

The ECG is usually abnormal and may demonstrate any of the following:
1. Left ventricular (LV) hypertrophy with the tallest QRS complex found in the midprecordial leads.
2. Pathological Q waves in leads II, III, AVF, or V_4 to V_6 or in any combination of these.
3. LAD (left axis deviation).
4. Features of Wolff-Parkinson-White (WPW) syndrome, including a short P-R interval and delta wave.

Echocardiography

Echocardiography demonstrates the following:
1. An increased thickness of the intraventricular septum relative to the left ventricular free wall, with a ratio of 1.3:1.0 or more at end-diastole.

2. During systole, an abnormal forward motion of the anterior mitral valve leaflet toward the septum.
3. At end-diastole, an abnormal anterior position of the mitral valve.

Chest X-ray

Chest X-ray demonstrates the following:
1. Normal heart size to enlarge LV.
2. Left atrial enlargement often seen.

Thallium-201 Myocardial Imaging

Thallium-201 imaging demonstrates differences in the relative thickness of the LV free wall and septum.

Cardiac Catheterization

Cardiac catheterization demonstrates the following:
1. Hypertrophy of the left ventricle with a small, irregular cavity at end-systole and exaggerated contraction.
2. In patients with obstruction, a pressure gradient in the left ventricle during systole on both sides of the obstruction.
3. Mitral regurgitation (in ± 50 per cent of patients).

COMPLICATIONS

Arrhythmia. This is due to atrial and ventricular hypertrophy or left ventricular stiffness.

Congestive Heart Failure. CHF results from left ventricular stiffness.

Pulmonary Hypertension. This is due to left ventricular stiffness.

Sudden Death. Death is caused by arrhythmia or obstruction.

MEDICAL AND NURSING MANAGEMENT

Beta-Blockers

Beta-blockers such as propranolol (Inderal) (20 to 60 mg PO q.i.d. up to 1 gm per day) or nadalol (Corgard) (80 to 240 mg q d) decrease the pressure gradient across the obstruction by reducing contractility and heart rate (thus ↑ left ventricular filling).

Calcium Channel Blockers

Calcium channel blockers such as verapamil are being used experimentally to relieve symptoms, and initial results appear favorable.

Rapid Conversion of Nonsinus Arrhythmias

Rapid conversion of nonsinus arrhythmias, often necessitating cardioversion, is important, as these patients need the contribution of atrial contraction to left ventricular filling.

Surgery

Surgery is indicated if medical management proves ineffective. It involves excision of a portion of the hypertrophied septum and occasionally mitral valve replacement.

Teaching of Patient and Family

Teaching is a necessity in the effective management of IHSS. The following areas should be stressed:

1. Avoid strenuous exercise.
2. Rest when tired.
3. Take medication as prescribed and understand its basic action and possible side effects.
4. Follow subacute bacterial endocarditis (SBE) precautions regarding any surgical procedure (includes dentistry) consisting of taking antibiotics (penicillin or erythromycin) before and for several days after the procedure.
5. Be aware of what factors aggravate and what factors relieve obstruction (see Table 16–4).
6. For the patient with angina, help in identification and alleviation of modifiable coronary risk factors such as smoking and weight control.
7. Offer opportunity for open discussion with the patient regarding the disease, attemping to aid him or her in coming to terms with a chronic condition.
8. Stress the importance of routine cardiological follow-ups.
9. Since IHSS carries with it the risk of sudden death, the patient's significant other should be encouraged to learn cardiopulmonary resuscitation (CPR).

Table 16-4. FACTORS AFFECTING OBSTRUCTION IN IDIOPATHIC HYPERTROPHIC SUBAORTIC STENOSIS (IHSS)

FACTORS THAT AGGRAVATE OBSTRUCTION	FACTORS THAT RELIEVE OBSTRUCTION
1. Tachycardia and nonsinus rhythms	1. ↑ Circulating volume
2. Strenuous exercise	2. Squatting position
3. Quick assumption of erect posture	3. "Shock" position—supine with legs elevated
4. ↑ Sympathetic stimulation	4. Beta-blockers: propranolol (Inderal) and nadolol (Corgard)
5. Valsalva maneuver	5. Methoxamine
6. Blood loss	6. Phenylephrine
7. Vigorous diuresis	7. Calcium channel blockers (verapamil)
8. Cardiac glycosides (digoxin)*	
9. Isoproterenol (Isuprel)	
10. Nitrates	
11. Paroxysms of coughing	

*Use of digoxin in patients with IHSS is controversial. Some authorities feel that its use is not detrimental in those patients who exhibit signs of congestive heart failure.

10. Because many patients with IHSS are asymptomatic, all first-degree family members of known IHSS patients should have echocardiographic screening, as they have a 50 per cent chance of having the disease.

Cor Pulmonale

DEFINITION

Cor pulmonale is hypertrophy and dilatation of the right ventricle secondary to lung disease rather than heart disease. Some degree of right-sided heart failure is usually present.

ETIOLOGY

Cor pulmonale results from conditions that cause increased vascular resistance in the lungs. Any pulmonary disease that affects ventilation, gas exchange or pulmonary vasculature (pulmonary hypertension) can cause cor pulmonale. These include chronic bronchitis or emphysema, pulmonary emboli, or pulmonary fibrosis.

PATHOPHYSIOLOGY

The right ventricle in comparison with the left is more compliant and thinner walled and better able to handle increased volume than pressure. Increased arteriolar resistance in the lungs and pulmonary hypertension increase the workload of the right ventricle and result in muscular hypertrophy and chamber dilatation of the right side of the heart. If pulmonary artery pressures become high enough, right-sided heart failure results.

PATIENT ASSESSMENT

Assessment includes evaluating the degree of lung damage and right-sided heart function.

Auscultation of the Heart

An S_4 gallop heard loudest at the left lower sternal border is often present and indicates right atrial enlargement and right ventricular failure.

Palpation of the PMI

If marked hypertrophy is present, a right ventricular heave or sternal lift can be palpated.

X-ray

On X-ray, an enlarged right heart silhouette is usually present.

Cardiac Monitoring

Atrial arrhythmias often result when the atrium is stretched. These include frequent PACs, atrial flutter and atrial fibrillation.

ECG Findings

Signs of right-sided strain or hypertrophy are indicated by changes in the right ventricular leads, aVR and V_1. There is a tall R wave in aVR. V_1 has a tall R wave, a slightly widened QRS, ST segment depression and an inverted T wave.

Monitoring for Heart Failure

Cor pulmonale patients should be observed for indications of progression to right heart failure. Signs include elevated central venous pressure (CVP), increased jugular vein distention and peripheral edema.

MANAGEMENT

Treatment is aimed at improving the underlying pulmonary disorder and correcting hypoxemia to reduce pulmonary resistance. Digitalis is seldom used for right-sided failure of cor pulmonale because of increased risk of toxicity. Diuretics are often used to effect unloading of the right heart.

SUGGESTED READINGS

Pericarditis

Fowler, N. O.: Physiology of cardiac tamponade and pulsus paradox. *Mod. Con. Cardiovasc. Dis.*, 47:115, 1978.

Moore, S. J.: Pericarditis after acute myocardial infarction. *Heart and Lung*, 8:551, 1979.

Ward, C.: Viral myopericarditis. *Chest, Heart and Stroke*, 3:10, 1978.

Myocarditis

Braunwald, E.: *Heart Disease*. Philadelphia, W. B. Saunders, 1980.

Ward, C.: Viral myopericarditis. *Chest, Heart, and Stroke*, 3:10, 1978.

Infective Endocarditis

Beeson, P. B., et al.: *Textbook of Medicine*, 15th ed. Philadelphia, W. B. Saunders, 1979.

Braunwald, E.: *Heart Disease*. Philadelphia, W. B. Saunders, 1980.

Conn, H. F. (ed.): *1982 Current Therapy*. Philadelphia, W. B. Saunders, 1982.

Conn, H. F., and Conn, R. B.: *Current Diagnosis*. Philadelphia, W. B. Saunders, 1980.

Eisenberg, M. S., and Copass, M. K.: *Manual of Emergency Medical Therapeutics*. Philadelphia, W. B. Saunders, 1978.

Sokolow, M., and McIlroy, M. B.: *Clinical Cardiology*. Los Altos, Lange Medical Publications, 1979.

Rheumatic Heart Disease

Alpert, J. S., and Rippe, J. M.: *Manual of Cardiovascular Diagnosis and Therapy*. Boston, Little, Brown, 1980.

Beeson, P. B., McDermott, W., and Wyngaarden, J. B.: *Cecil Textbook of Medicine*, 15th ed., Vol. I, Philadelphia, W. B. Saunders, 1979.

Conn, H. F.: *1982 Current Therapy*. Philadelphia, W. B. Saunders, 1982.

Conn, H. F., and Conn, R. B.: *Current Diagnosis*. Philadelphia, W. B. Saunders, 1980, pp. 338–345.

Isselbacher, K. J., et al.: *Harrison's Principles of Internal Medicine*, 9th ed. New York, McGraw-Hill, 1980.

Wenger, N. K., Hurst, J. W., and McIntyre, M. C.: *Cardiology for Nurses*. New York, McGraw-Hill, 1980.

Cardiomyopathy

Breu, C. S., et al.: Treatment of patients with congestive cardiomyopathy during hospitalization: A case study. *Heart and Lung*, 11:229, 1982.

Dracup, K.: Unraveling the mysteries of cardiomyopathy. *Nursing '79*, 9:84, 1979.

Haughey, C.: Alcoholic cardiomyopathy: abstinence makes the heart grow stronger. *Nursing '80* 10:9, 1980.

Hurst, J. W.: The Heart. New York, McGraw-Hill, 1978.

Meyer, R., and Morris, D.: Alcoholic cardiomyopathy: a nursing approach. *Nurs. Res.*, 26:422, 1977.

Sokolow, M., et al.: *Clinical Cardiology*. Los Altos, Lange Medical Publications, 1979.

Idiopathic Hypertrophic Subaortic Stenosis (IHSS)

Arobogast, R. C., and White, R.: Idiopathic hypertrophic subaortic stenosis. *Am. Fam. Phys.*, 24:97, 1981.

Braunwald, E.: *Heart Disease*. Philadelphia, W. B. Saunders, 1980.

Egoville, B. B.: IHSS. *Nursing '80*, 10:51, 1980.

Hurst, J. W.: *The Heart*. New York, McGraw-Hill, 1978.

Cor Pulmonale

Ferrer, M. I.: Management of patients with cor pulmonale. *Med. Clin. North Am.*, 63:251, 1979.

Hartman, R. B.: Pulmonary heart disease: pathophysiology, diagnostic steps and therapy. *Postgrad. Med.*, 66(3):58, 1979.

Meador, B.: Why COPD can end in heart failure. . . . and what you can do about it?" *RN*, 43:64, 1980.

IV

SPECIFIC MEDICAL THERAPIES

17

MEDICATIONS COMMONLY USED IN CCU

Medications presented in this chapter are categorized according to their *main* actions, although some may have more than one clinical use. For easy reference, the major categories as well as drugs within each category are arranged alphabetically, except the miscellaneous group, which is listed at the end.

The content of this chapter is focused on cardiac patients. Therefore, noncardiac indications, actions and dosages are omitted. Since most of the cardiac drugs are either eliminated from the kidneys or detoxified in the liver, caution should be used in patients with decreased hepatic or renal function. The recommended dosages are for adults and may vary according to the physician's preference.

The major categories included are as follows:

1. Antiarrhythmic drugs (Table 17–1)
2. Anticoagulant drugs (Table 17–2)
3. Antiplatelet drugs (Table 17–3)
4. Autonomic drugs (Table 17–4)
5. Calcium channel blockers (Table 17–5)
6. Cardiotonic drugs (Table 17–6)
7. Diuretics (Table 17–7)
8. Vasodilators (Table 17–8)
9. Miscellaneous (diazepam, meperidine, morphine, potassium, sodium bicarbonate) (Table 17–9)

Table 17–1. ANTIARRHYTHMIC DRUGS

DRUG	INDICATIONS	ACTIONS	USUAL DOSAGE	SIDE EFFECTS OR COMPLICATIONS	NURSING CONSIDERATIONS
Bretylium tosylate (Bretylol)	Emergency treatment of life-threatening ventricular arrhythmias when other drugs are ineffective	Mechanisms not well established; observations made: Little effect on automaticity	*IV:* Push: in ventricular fibrillation: 5–10 mg/kg; may repeat in 15–30 minutes	Hypotension (in 50 per cent of patients) accompanied by vertigo, dizziness and syncope	Monitor cardiac rhythms; may see initial worsening of arrhythmia.
		↑Ventricular fibrillation threshold	Other use: dilute 1 amp (500 mg/10 ml) in 50 ml D₅W; give 5–10 mg/kg over 10–20 minutes q 6 hours	Severe nausea and vomiting	Patient should remain in supine position during injection.
		Initially increases, then inhibits the release of norepinephrine	Drip: 1–2 mg/minute	May transiently increase heart rate and blood pressure	IV push should be very slow.
		Positive inotropic and chronotropic effects	*IM:* No dilution		IM sites should be changed.
			5–10 mg/kg q 6–8 hours		May potentiate digitalis toxicity.
			Onset within minutes with IV use		Hypotension effect may be augmented when used with diuretics and vasodilators.
			Half-life: 6–10 hours		

Table continued on following page

Table 17-1. ANTIARRHYTHMIC DRUGS (Continued)

DRUG	INDICATIONS	ACTIONS	USUAL DOSAGE	SIDE EFFECTS OR COMPLICATIONS	NURSING CONSIDERATIONS
Disopyramide (Norpace)	Ventricular arrhythmias	Same as quinidine and procainamide except that its anticholinergic effect is stronger	*PO:* Loading dose: 200–300 mg Maintenance dose: 100–200 mg q 6 hours Peaks in ½ to 3 hours Half-life; 6 hours	Dry mouth, urinary hesitancy and retention Anorexia, nausea and vomiting Myocardial depression Heart blocks Hypotension and even cardiogenic shock	Monitor cardiac rhythms. Use with caution in patients with enlarged prostate, congestive heart failure (CHF) and heart block.
Lidocaine (Xylocaine)	Ventricular ectopic beats Ventricular arrhythmias Prophylaxis for ventricular fibrillation (VF) in MI patients	↓ Automaticity of Purkinje fibers ↓ Action potential duration (APD) more than effective refractory period (ERP) and prevents completion of the re-entry circuit of a tachyarrhythmia	*IV:* Push: 50–100 mg (up to 400 mg/hour) Drip: 2–4 mg/minute Onset: in 45 to 90 seconds Effects last 20 minutes after IV push and 2 hours after discontinuation of IV drip	Early signs: lethargy, dizziness, muscle twitching, blurred and double vision, sweating, slurred speech Seizures → coma Heart blocks Sinus arrest	Cardiac rhythm should be monitored constantly on scope. Contraindicated in patients with heart blocks. Caution in patients with bradycardia. Dosage should be decreased as soon as toxic effects appear.

Drug	Action	Uses	Dosage	Side effects	Nursing considerations
Phenytoin (Dilantin)	↓ Automaticity ↓ APD more than ERP, similar to lidocaine	Digitalis-induced arrhythmias More effective for ventricular than atrial arrhythmias Tricyclic antidepressant overdose-induced arrhythmias	IV: 50–100 mg over 5–10 minutes q 5 minutes up to 1000 mg PO: Loading, 1 gm Maintenance, 100 mg q.i.d. Peaks in 48–96 hours Half-life: 13–24 hours	Nystagmus, ataxia, lethargy, nausea, vertigo, rashes, pseudolymphoma, megaloblastic anemia, peripheral neuropathy, hyperglycemia and seizures Rapid IV injection may cause hypotension, 1:1 conduction in atrial flutter, respiratory arrest; ventricular fibrillation and cardiac arrest	Monitor cardiac rhythms and blood pressure (BP) during IV injection, which should be extremely slow. Injection in smaller vein may cause discomfort and phlebitis. Use with caution in patients with bradycardia and heart blocks. Reduce dose when oral anticoagulants are used. This drug is incompatible with levarterenal bitartrate (Levophed).
Procainamide (Pronestyl, Procan SR)	Same as quinidine	Ventricular arrhythmias Ventricular arrhythmias refractory to lidocaine or used in conjection with lidocaine Atrial arrhythmias (less frequent)	IV: Push: 100 mg in 1–3 minutes, q 1 hour Drip: 100 mg (not to exceed 1000 mg); loading dose followed with 1–4 mg/minute Effect: immediate PO: 250–500 mg q 3–4 hours	Anorexia, nausea and vomiting Dizziness, giddiness, mental depression, hallucinations, psychosis Worsens CHF Agranulocytosis Lupus-like syndrome (reversible)	Monitor cardiac rhythms, especially during IV injection. Observe for and report excessive widening of QRS and Q-T. This drug is contraindicated in patients with atrioventricular (AV) blocks. Obtain frequent blood counts for detecting agranulocytosis. Use extreme caution during IV push.

Table continued on following page

Table 17-1. ANTIARRHYTHMIC DRUGS (Continued)

DRUG	INDICATIONS	ACTIONS	USUAL DOSAGE	SIDE EFFECTS OR COMPLICATIONS	NURSING CONSIDERATIONS
Procainamide (Pronestyl, Procan SR) *Continued*			Sustained release: 500–1000 mg q 6 hours Oral effect peaks in 45–75 minutes Half-life: 3–4 hours Duration of sustained release form can last for 8 hours	Hypotension and cardiovascular collapse possibly caused by IV injection	
Quinidine: 1. Quinidine sulfate (Cin-Quin, Quinora, Quinidex)	Atrial flutter and fibrillation—for conversion or prophylaxis after cardioversion Atrial and ventricular premature beats	↓ Automaticity, excitability, contractility, and vagal tone ↑ Effective refractory period (ERP), action potential duration (APD) and conduction time	*IV:* Quinidine gluconate, 10 ml (800-mg vial) diluted in 50 ml D_5W; 80 to 100 mg in 5 minutes	Nausea, vomiting, diarrhea, vertigo, light-headedness, tinnitis, tremor, headache, blurred vision and abdominal cramps	Monitor cardiac rhythm. Closely observe the patient during IV injection. Observe for and report extreme prolongation of QRS and Q-T.

		PO:	Sinus and/or AV block	Give with meals if possible to lessen the GI symptoms.
2. Quinidine gluconate (Quinaglute, also in injection form)	PAT	Quinidine sulfate, 200–400 mg q 6 hours	Worsens CHF	Digitalis is usually started before quinidine in atrial fibrillation and flutter patients who have rapid ventricular rate.
	Ventricular tachycardia	Sustained release quinidine sulfate (Quinidex), 300 mg q 8–12 hours	Quinidine syncope: hypotension, ventricular tachycardia (VT), sudden death and other hypersensitivity reactions (fever, rashes, hepatitis, thrombocytopenic purpura)	Check serum level as needed.
3. Quinidine polygalacturonate (Cardioquin)		Quinaglute, 324 mg q 8–12 hours		A sensitivity test may be given before first dose.
		Cardioquin, 275 mg q 6 hours		Owing to potentiated digitalis effect, a decreased maintenance digitalis dose should be considered.
		Sulfate: peaks in 60–90 minutes		Use of IV quinidine is contraindicated for VT secondary to digital toxicity.
		Half-life: 6 hours		
		Gluconate: peaks in 3–4 hours; release slowly (8–12 hours) in gastrointestinal (GI) tract		

Table 17-2. ANTICOAGULANT DRUGS

DRUG	INDICATIONS	ACTIONS	USUAL DOSAGE	SIDE EFFECTS OR COMPLICATIONS	NURSING CONSIDERATIONS
Heparin sodium	Short-term anticoagulation	Neutralizes thrombin, preventing conversion of fibrinogen to fibrin	For full anticoagulation, individualized dose is determined by whole-blood clotting time (therapeutic anticoagulation is 2–3 times control value)	Hemorrhage	As an antidote use 1% protamine sulfate solution via slow IV injection.
	Treatment of venous thrombosis, pulmonary emboli	Delays activation of fibrin stabilizing factor		Hematoma if given IM	Do not give IM.
	Prevention of mural thrombi formation due to atrial fibrillation		*IV:* Push: loading dose, 10,000 units; maintenance 5000–10,000 units, q 4–6 hours	Hypersensitivity reaction: fever, chills, urticaria	Watch for any signs of bleeding (especially, mucous membranes) or excessive bruising.
	Prophylaxis for thromboembolism following MI			Acute, reversible thrombocytopenia	
	Pulmonary emboli		Drip: loading dose, 5000 units followed by drip to total 20,000–40,000 units per day	Osteoporosis, associated with long-term therapy	
			Onset: immediate		

Drug	Action	Use	Dose	Side Effects/Toxicity	Nursing Implications
			SQ: Loading dose, 10,000–20,000 units; Maintenance, 8000–10,000 units q 8 hours; Prophylactic low dose, 5000 units q 8 hours; Duration; depends on route, usually 4–6 hours		
Crystalline warfarin sodium (Coumadin)	Inhibits synthesis of prothrombin in the liver (competes with vitamin K) and thus interferes with fibrin formation and growth of thrombi	Long-term anticoagulation; Treatment of venous thrombosis, pulmonary emboli; Prevention of venous thrombosis and mural thrombi formation due to atrial fibrillation and systemic emboli	Dose individualized and determined by obtaining periodic prothrombin times (therapeutic anticoagulation is 1½–2½ times normal prothrombin level) PO: Loading dose, 20–60 mg given once only; Maintenance dose, 2–10 mg daily; Onset: 1–9 hours	Hemorrhage	As an antidote use vitamin K, fresh blood, plasma. Observe for and teach patient to recognize signs of bleeding, especially from mucous membranes; watch for "tarry stools," "coffee ground emesis," nosebleed, blood in urine. Caution patient against participating in contact sports (bruising). Encourage patient to carry ID card stating that he or she is on anticoagulants.

Table continued on following page

Table 17–2. ANTICOAGULANT DRUGS (Continued)

DRUG	INDICATIONS	ACTIONS	USUAL DOSAGE	SIDE EFFECTS OR COMPLICATIONS	NURSING CONSIDERATIONS

Crystalline warfarin sodium (Coumadin) *Continued*			Peak: 36–72 hours
			
			Duration: 4–5 days
			
			Half-life: 2½ days
			
			Also available in parenteral form, but PO route is preferred
					Caution patient not to take any other medications without first consulting physician.
					
					Drugs that ↑ anticoagulation effects of Coumadin are as follows:
					  Salicylates
					  Antibiotics
					  Anabolic steroids
					  Phenylbutazone
					  Thyroid extract
					  Cholestyramine
					  Oral hypoglycemic agents
					  Alcohol (acute ingestion of)
					
					Drugs that ↓ anticoagulation effects of Coumadin are as follows:
					  Diuretics
					  Corticosteroids
					  Meprobamate
					  Estrogens
					  Barbiturates
					  Antacids
					  Allopurinol
					  Alcohol (chronic ingestion of)

Table 17-3. ANTIPLATELET DRUGS

DRUG	INDICATIONS	ACTIONS	USUAL DOSAGE	SIDE EFFECTS OR COMPLICATIONS	NURSING CONSIDERATIONS
Dipyridamole (Persantine)	Prevention of arterial thrombosis	Interferes with platelet aggregation	*PO:* 50 mg 2-3 times a day, usually taken with salicylates	Nausea Dizziness, headache Weakness Flushing Hypersensitivity frequently seen in patients with hypersensitivity to salicylates	This drug is also a potent coronary vasodilator, but the value of its use in treatment of angina has yet to be proved.
Sulfinpyrazone (Anturane)	Prevention of arterial thrombosis ↓ incidence of sudden death post MI	Interferes with normal platelet function and inhibits synthesis of prostaglandins and thromboxane	*PO:* 200 mg 1-4 times daily	Contraindicated in patients with GI inflammation or ulcer or in patients with blood dyscrasia Renal colic GI disturbances Rash	Give this drug with food, milk or antacids. This drug may potentiate sulfa drugs and insulin.

Table 17–4. AUTONOMIC DRUGS

DRUG	INDICATIONS	ACTIONS	USUAL DOSAGE	SIDE EFFECTS OR COMPLICATIONS	NURSING CONSIDERATIONS
Agonists *Alpha-agonists* Methoxamine (Vasoxyl)	Counteract severe hypotension caused by anesthesia and drug reactions Supraventricular tachycardia	Vasoconstriction causes ↑ blood pressure and peripheral vascular resistance Slows AV conduction	*IV:* 3–10 mg slowly Onset: immediate Duration: 1 hour *IM:* 10–20 mg Onset: 15 minutes Duration: 90 minutes	Severe bradycardia, headache, urinary urgency, projectile vomiting, pilomotor response	Monitor heart rate and blood pressure. Keep atropine on hand for reflex bradycardia. Use with caution in patients with myocardial infarction, CHF, hyperthyroidism.
Phenylephrine (Neo-Synephrine)	Paroxysmal atrial tachycardia Hypotensive crisis Antidote for chlorpromazine (Thorazine)-induced hypotension	Sympathomimetic—increases stroke volume and blood pressure	*IV:* Push: 0.1–0.5 mg over 1 minute, (dilute 1 mg in 9 ml of IV solution) Drip: 10 mg in 250 ml D₅W or NS and titrate	Reflex bradycardia, ventricular irritability, hypertensive crisis, tingling of extremities	Phentolamine (Regitine) is the agent of choice to reverse a severe hypertensive response. This drug is potentiated by other sympathomimetics, tricyclic antidepressants, MAO inhibitors.

Drug	Indications	Actions	Dosage	Side effects	Nursing considerations
Beta-agonists Isoproterenol (Isuprel)	Cardiogenic shock with ↑ peripheral vascular resistance; Septic shock (as an adjunct); Advanced AV block; Idioventricular rhythms; Bronchospasms	Cardiac stimulant (positive inotropic and chronotropic effects); ↑ Systolic BP; Peripheral vasodilation; ↑ AV conduction; Bronchial smooth muscle relaxation	Onset: 15 seconds; Duration: 15 minutes; SQ/IM: 2–5 mg q 10–15 minutes; duration 1–2 hours; *IV Drip:* 1–2 mg in 500 ml D$_5$W; titrate for effects—average = 1–8 mcg/kg/minute	Tachycardia, palpitations, hypotension, ventricular irritability, angina, cardiac arrest	Monitor blood pressure every 2–3 minutes. This drug is incompatible with alkaline solutions. Closely monitor blood pressure and heart rhythm. This may be used as an antagonist to propranolol. Use with caution in patients with coronary insufficiency, hypovolemia, hypokalemia, diabetes or tachycardia.
Beta- and alpha-agonists Dobutamine	Cardiogenic shock with ↑ peripheral vascular resistance	Works selectively on beta-1 receptors; Very mild alpha effects; ↑ Contractility; Slight chronotropic effects	*IV:* Drip: 250–500 mg in 500 ml D$_5$W; 2.5–10 mcg/kg/minute; Titrate for effects	Marked tachycardia, nausea, headache, palpitations, shortness of breath and anginal pain	This agent is similar to dopamine except that there is no renal artery vasodilation. Closely monitor heart rate, rhythm, blood pressure and urine output.

Table continued on following page

Table 17–4. AUTONOMIC DRUGS (Continued)

DRUG	INDICATIONS	ACTIONS	USUAL DOSAGE	SIDE EFFECTS OR COMPLICATIONS	NURSING CONSIDERATIONS
Dobutamine *Continued*		Enhances AV conduction High dose (>15 mcg/kg/minute) produces vasodilation	Half-life: 2 minutes		This agent is contraindicated in patients with ventricular tachycardia or idiopathic subaortic stenosis.
Dopamine HCl (Intropin)	Shock associated with myocardial infarction, sepsis, congestive heart failure and renal failure	↑ Systolic blood pressure ↑ Cardiac output ↑ Renal blood flow (in doses < 20 mcg/kg/minute) ↑ Peripheral vascular resistance in doses > 5–10 mcg/kg/minute	*IV Drip:* 200–400 mg in 250–500 ml D_5W Titrate for effects: 2–5 mcg/kg/minute Effects last 10 minutes (See infusion dose chart in Appendix 6)	Tachycardia, headache, precordial pain, nausea, vomiting	Correct hypovolemia prior to using. Monitor heart rate, blood pressure and urine output (to titrate dosage). Dosages of > 20 mcg/kg/minute → ↓ renal blood flow (alpha effects). This is often used in conjunction with nitroprusside to maximize cardiac function. This drug is incompatible with alkaline solutions

Epinephrine (Adrenalin)	Cardiac arrest: asystole or fine ventricular fibrillation	Potent vasoconstrictor, ↑ peripheral vascular resistance	*Cardiac arrest:* IV: 5–10 ml (1:10,000); repeat q 5 minutes as needed (may give intracardiac or intratracheal)	Weakness, vertigo, anxiety, psychosis, ventricular irritability, pulmonary edema, hypertension	Extravasation may cause necrosis (phentolamine will reverse it.)
					This drug is contraindicated in patients with pheochromocytoma or tachyarrhythmias or in those on MAO inhibitors.
	Stokes-Adams syndrome	Positive chronotropic and inotropic effects	Onset: immediate		Phentolamine (Regitine) can reverse severe hypertensive response.
	Anaphylactic shock	Bronchial smooth muscle relaxation	*Anaphylaxis: SQ or IM:* 0.1 to 0.5 ml (1:1000)		Neostigmine is used to treat other toxic effects.
					This agent is incompatible in alkaline solutions.
	Bronchospasm	Histamine antidote			This drug is contraindicated in patients with hypertension, glaucoma and hyperthyroidism and in those who are digitalized.

Table continued on following page

Table 17-4. AUTONOMIC DRUGS (Continued)

DRUG	INDICATIONS	ACTIONS	USUAL DOSAGE	SIDE EFFECTS OR COMPLICATIONS	NURSING CONSIDERATIONS
Levarterenol bitartrate (Levophed, Norepinephrine)	Severe hypotension	Potent vasoconstriction, ↑ peripheral vascular resistance Mild ↑ in heart rate Coronary artery dilation ↓ Renal blood flow	*IV Drip:* 4–8 mg in 500 ml D₅W Titrate for effects Average: 2–4 mcg/kg/minute	Tissue necrosis and sloughing if infiltrated ↑ Myocardial ischemia Bradycardia Severe hypertension	Phentolamine (Regitine), 5–10 mg in 10–15 ml saline, injected into infiltrated area will prevent local necrosis. Use with caution in hemorrhagic shock (replace volume first). Check BP q 2 minutes initially and q 5 minutes thereafter. Use with caution in patients on MAO inhibitors. This drug is incompatible with whole blood, heparin sodium, sodium bicarbonate and phenytoin (Dilantin).
Metaraminol bitartrate (Aramine)	Acute hypotension Supraventricular tachycardia	Vasoconstriction—↑ peripheral vascular resistance ↑ Blood pressure ↑ Myocardial contractility	*IV Drip:* 15–100 mg in 500 ml D₅W Titrate for effects Effects begin in 1–2 minutes	Hypertension, ventricular irritability, reflex bradycardia and tissue sloughing (if infiltrated)	This agent is incompatible with alkaline solutions. This drug is contraindicated in conjunction with cyclopropane or halothane anesthesia.

Antagonists
Alpha-antagonists

Phenoxybenzamine (Dibenzyline)	Peripheral vasodilator Increases blood flow to skin and viscera Pheochromocytoma Vasospastic peripheral vascular disease (i.e., Raynaud's syndrome)	*PO:* Initially 10 mg/day for 4 days, then 20–60 mg/day 2 weeks needed for optimum blood level	Nasal congestion, hypotension, tachycardia, inhibited ejaculation	For hypotension effects, levarterenol (Levophed) may help. This drug is contraindicated in patients with cerebral or coronary atherosclerosis or hypotension.
Phentolamine (Regitine)	Vasodilation, ↓ peripheral vascular resistance Prevent tissue necrosis from levarterenol infiltration Possible use in shock with prolonged vasoconstriction Pheochromocytoma	To prevent *tissue sloughing*, 5–10 mg in 10 ml saline and inject into area of infiltration within 1–2 hours *IV:* 5–20 mg, rapidly *IV Drip:* 100–500 mg per liter, titrate for effect *IM:* 5–20 mg Onset: instant	Acute hypotension, cardiac arrhythmias, vertigo, gastrointestinal distress	Monitor blood pressure and pulse prior to and during administration. Histamine-like effects may potentiate peptic ulcers. Do not reverse phentolamine-induced shock with epinephrine.

Table continued on following page

Table 17–4. AUTONOMIC DRUGS (Continued)

DRUG	INDICATIONS	ACTIONS	USUAL DOSAGE	SIDE EFFECTS OR COMPLICATIONS	NURSING CONSIDERATIONS
Prazosin (Minipress)	Hypertension	Arterial vasodilation causes ↓ peripheral vascular resistance	*PO:* 1–2 mg q.i.d Peaks in 3 hours	Postural hypotension, vertigo, syncope, drowsiness, palpitations, nausea, rash, urinary frequency, nervousness, diaphoresis	Patients should be monitored closely, as postural hypotension and syncope may occur 30 to 90 minutes after dose is initiated.
Beta-antagonists Propranolol (Inderal)	Angina pectoris	Negative chronotropic and inotropic effects	*IV Push:* 2–10 mg slowly (give ½ mg as test dose, then 1 mg q 3–4 minutes up to 10 mg)	Hypotension, congestive heart failure, AV block, AV dissociation, cardiac arrest, bronchoconstriction and hypoglycemia (in insulin-dependent people)	*Do not withdraw* abruptly (exacerbates myocardial ischemia).
	Tachyarrhythmia (especially PAT)	↓ Myocardial oxygen needs			Closely monitor ECG and blood pressure during IV administration.
	Ventricular arrhythmias due to digitalis toxicity	Slows AV conduction	Onset: 1–3 minutes		This agent is contraindicated in patients with congestive heart failure, asthma, bradycardia or advanced AV block, hypoglycemia.
	Hypertension	Antagonizes both beta 1 and beta 2 effects (nonselective)	Peaks: 10–15 minutes		
	Idiopathic hypertrophic subaortic stenosis (IHSS)		*PO:* 20–250 mg/day in divided doses		Instruct the patient on home use (pulse-taking, daily weights).
	↓ Risk of reinfarction		Peaks: 1–1½ hours Half life: 2–3 hours		Toxic effects are reversed by isoproterenol or dopamine.

Drug	Uses	Actions	Dosage	Side effects	Nursing considerations
Metoprolol (Lopressor)	Same as propranolol	Same as propranol except that it selectively antagonizes beta 1 effect	PO: 100–450 mg/day Peaks: 90 minutes Half-life: 3 hours	Same as propranolol but no respiratory distress	Nursing considerations are the same as for propranolol.
Nadolol (Corgard)	Chronic angina pectoris Hypertension Reverse isoproterenol-induced tachycardia ↓ Risk of reinfarction	Negative chronotropic effects ↓ AV conduction ↓ Myocardial oxygen needs Suppression of renin secretion Nonselective beta effects Three times more potent than propranolol	PO: 80–320 mg q d Peak: 3–4 hours Duration: 20–24 hours	Vertigo, gastrointestinal distress, bronchospasm, hypotension, congestive heart failure, hypoglycemia, rash and hallucinations	Nursing considerations are the same as for propranolol. Nadolol is longer acting than propranolol.
Timolol mallate (Blocadren)	Angina pectoris Antihypertensive ↓ Risk of reinfarction ↓ Size of infarction	Nonselective beta effects Six times more potent than propranolol ↓ Myocardial contractility ↓ Heart rate	PO: 10–30 mg b.i.d. (7-day interval between dose increases)	Hypotension, congestive heart failure, bradycardia, cardiogenic shock Raynaud's syndrome Nausea, vomiting, diarrhea	Nursing considerations are the same as for propranolol.

Table continued on following page

Table 17–4. AUTONOMIC DRUGS (Continued)

DRUG	INDICATIONS	ACTIONS	USUAL DOSAGE	SIDE EFFECTS OR COMPLICATIONS	NURSING CONSIDERATIONS
Timolol mallate (Blocarden) Continued		Slows AV conduction ↓ Myocardial oxygen needs		Impotence, dysuria Rash, hyperpigmentation Nightmares, psychoses	
Parasympatholytic Atropine sulfate	Symptomatic bradycardia, including heart block	Anticholinergic ↑ heart rate ↑ AV conduction	IV Push: 0.5–1.0 mg up to 2 mg Repeat q 4–6 hours Rapid onset	Flushing, nervousness, urinary hesitancy, psychosis, dry mouth, visual blurring, fever, tachycardia	This drug is incompatible in solutions with sodium bicarbonate and epinephrine. Atropine poisoning is reversed by neostigmine methylsulfate.
Parasympathomimetic Edrophonium chloride (Tensilon)	Paroxysmal atrial tachycardia (PAT) Reversal of effects from tubocurarine and curare	Blocks acetylcholinesterase ↓ Heart rate	IV Push: 2–10 mg over 2–4 minutes Rapid onset Short duration (10 minutes)	Cardiac arrest, vomiting, seizures, respiratory distress, laryngospasm, urinary frequency, gastrointestinal distress	This drug prolongs the effects of succinylcholine (Anectine). This is not the first choice in treating paroxysmal atrial tachycardia.

Sympatholytic Methyldopa (Aldomet)	Moderate-to-severe hypertension Renal hypertension	↓ Peripheral vascular resistance ↓ Blood pressure	*IV:* 250–500 mgm q 6–8 hours Slow onset: 4–6 hours *PO:* 250 mgm once or twice daily Onset: 6–12 hours	Headache, vertigo, orthostatic hypotension, syncope, anemia, fever, sedation, depression, nasal congestion, sodium and water retention hemolytic anemia and liver disorders.	Monitor daily weights and intake and output. Urine may appear darker or blue. Caution patient to arise slowly. It should not be used for patients with liver dysfunctions.
Guanethidine sulfate (Ismelin)	Moderate-to-severe hypertension	Selective blockade of efferent peripheral sympathetic pathways Gradual ↓ in blood pressure and peripheral vascular resistance Slight ↓ in cardiac output	*PO:* 10 mg, initially, increase by 10 mg q 5–7 days Average dose: 10–50 mg/day	Vertigo, fatigue, bradycardia, diarrhea, edema and congestive heart failure, impotence, depression	Observe for postural hypotension. Measure daily weights. Side effects are dose-related. This drug is often given concurrently with thiazide diuretics.
Reserpine (Serpasil)	Hypertension	Depletes norepinephrine from central adrenergic nerve endings ↓ Peripheral vascular resistance ↓ Blood pressure	*IM:* 0.5–1.0 mg, then 2–4 mg q 3 hours *PO:* 0.5 mg/day for 2 weeks, then 0.1–0.25 mg/day	Drowsiness, vertigo, severe depression, nervousness, dysuria, nasal congestion, weight gain, edema, arrhythmias, abdominal cramps	Watch for depression. Concurrent use of digitalis and quinidine ↑ chance of arrhythmias. Avoid use in patients with history of depression or suicide attempts or in those taking MAO inhibitors.

Table 17–5. CALCIUM CHANNEL BLOCKERS

DRUG	INDICATIONS	ACTIONS	USUAL DOSAGE	SIDE EFFECTS OR COMPLICATIONS	NURSING CONSIDERATIONS
Nifedipine (Procardia)	Antianginal agent; prophylactic treatment of angina pectoris and Prinzmetal's variant angina	Slow calcium channel blocker	*Oral or sublingual:*	Headache	Occasionally, ischemic symptoms are enhanced by hypotension.
		Inhibits cellular uptake of calcium ions in vascular smooth muscle	Initial dose: 10 mg	Dizziness	An average reduction in mean arterial pressure of 36 mm Hg has been reported. It occurs 5 minutes after sublingual route and 20 minutes after oral route.
			Maintenance: 10–30 mg t.i.d.	Palpitations	
		Direct dilatory effect on coronary and peripheral vessels	Maximal dose: 180 mg/day	Weakness	
	Hypertension			Nausea	
		Mild coronary vasodilation → increased coronary blood low	Onset: Oral, 20 minutes	Flushing	This drug has enhanced effectiveness when used with beta-blockers.
	Acute myocardial infarction		Sublingual 5 minutes	Hypotension	
		Potent coronary artery antispasmodic	Peak: 1–2 hours	Side effects similar to those of nitroglycerin	
			Half-life: 4–5 hours		
		Reduction of systolic and diastolic blood pressure			
		Decreases cardiac workload			

Verapamil HCl (Calan, Isoptin)	Supraventricular tachyarrhythmias, including those of Wolff-Parkinson-White (WPW) and Lown-Ganong-Levine (LGL) syndromes	Inhibits Ca^{++} flux in the slow calcium channels of vascular smooth muscle	*IV:* Initial dose: IV bolus of 5–10 mg over 2–8 minutes	*Adverse reactions:* Hypotension
	Drug of choice for PAT	Prolongs AV node refractoriness	Repeat dose: 10 mg (0.15 mgm/kg) 30 minutes after first dose if response is not adequate	Rapid ventricular rate in atrial flutter or fibrillation in patients with WPW
	Control of rapid ventricular rate in atrial flutter or fibrillation	Reduces myocardial contractility	Onset: Less than 5 minutes	Extreme bradycardia or asystole
	Prinzmetal's angina	Dilates coronary and systemic vessels (less than nifedipine)	Peak: 3–5 minutes	The P-R is lengthened.
	Acute myocardial ischemia		Half-life: <30 minutes	This drug has no effect on R-R, QRS or Q-T.
	IHSS (under investigation)		Duration: 2–5 hours	Patients should be monitored to detect adverse reactions.
			Oral: 80–160 mg q 8 hours	Contraindications are as follows: Severe hypotension Cardiogenic shock Severe heart failure Patients on propranolol therapy Sick sinus syndrome
			Peak: 3–4 hours	
			Half-life: 3–7 hours	

Table 17–6. CARDIOTONIC DRUGS

DRUG	INDICATIONS	ACTIONS	USUAL DOSAGE	SIDE EFFECTS OR COMPLICATIONS	NURSING CONSIDERATIONS
Calcium chloride, 10% solution	Cardiac standstill, especially electromechanical dissociation Weak or ineffectual myocardial contractions Antagonizes toxicity of hyperkalemia	Activates contractile machinery Increases automaticity and impulse propagation	*IV Push:* 2.5–5 ml of 10% solution (100 mg/ml or 1.4 m Eq per ml); 250–500 mg	Irritating to tissue Rapid injection may cause vasodilation, decreased blood pressure, arrhythmias and cardiac arrest	Calcium should be given cautiously, if at all, to digitalized patients. Should be injected slowly (0.7–1.5 m Eq/min). Rapid infusion can cause severe bradycardia or sinus arrest. Extravasation into the tissue can cause necrosis. Precipitation occurs in IV tubing if given simultaneously with NaHCO$_3$.
Calcium gluconate, 10% solution	Same as calcium chloride	Same as calcium chloride	*IV Push:* 10 ml of 10% solution (4.8 m Eq)	Same as calcium chloride	Nursing considerations are the same as for calcium chloride.
Digitalis Digitoxin (Crystodigin)	Same as digoxin	Same as digoxin but longer lasting	*Digitalization:* 1.2–1.6 mg in divided doses *Maintenance:* 0.05–0.2 mg/day *IV Push:* Onset: 25 min–2 hr Peak: 4–12 hours	*Toxicity:* Plasma level >3.4 (therapeutic, 1.4–2.6); symptoms the same as for digoxin except that they may last longer	Nursing considerations are the same as for digoxin.

Digoxin (Lanoxin)	Rapid atrial fibrillation and flutter	Increases myocardial contractility (inotropic effect)	*PO:* Onset: 30 minutes–2 hours Peak: 4–12 hours Duration: 5 days to 2 weeks	*Toxicity:* Plasma level >2.4 (therapeutic, 0.8–1.6); side effects include anorexia, nausea, vomiting, diarrhea, blurred or "yellow" vision with haloes around objects, abdominal pain, restlessness, mental confusion, slow pulse rate, any arrhythmias but especially ventricular bigeminy, PAT with block	First-degree AV block is common. Digitalis has a very narrow therapeutic range, predisposing to toxicity.
	Atrial tachycardias, especially PAT	Vagal effect on sinus and AV node, which slows the heart rate and AV conduction	*Digitalization:* 1.5–2 mg *Maintenance:* 0.125–0.5 mg/day		Decreased serum potassium intensifies action of digitalis. Digitalis dosage may be reduced if quinidine is added.
	Congestive heart failure, especially low-output failure	Increases automaticity of myocardium	*IV Push:* Onset: 15–30 minutes Peak: 1–5 hours		Digitalized patients should not be given calcium except during an emergency.
			PO: Onset: 1–2 hours Peak: 6–8 hours Duration: 36 hours		Digitalis is contraindicated in heart block, severe myocarditis, IHSS. Patient teaching includes: Taking of pulse Daily weights Recognition of symptoms of CHF Recognition of symptoms of toxicity

Table 17–7. DIURETICS

DRUG	INDICATIONS	ACTIONS	USUAL DOSAGE	SIDE EFFECTS OR COMPLICATIONS	NURSING CONSIDERATIONS
Aldosterone antagonists Spironolactone (Aldactone)	Refractory edema Mild hypertension Frequently used in conjunction with other diuretics	Antagonizes aldosterone by competing for receptor sites	*Oral only:* 100 mg/day	Hyperkalemia Hypovolemia Gastrointestinal symptoms Gynecomastia	Electrolytes should be monitored.
Benzothiadiazides Chlorothiazide (Diuril)	Edema of CHF Mild hypertension Potentiates other antihypertensives	Inhibits reabsorption of sodium and chloride in distal tubule Augments potassium excretion Does not directly affect acid-base balance	500 mg–2 gm/day in 1–2 doses *IV Push:* Onset: 15 minutes Peak: 30 minutes Duration: 2 hours *Oral:* Duration 6–12 hours	Clinical toxicity rare Potassium depletion	Use all thiazides with caution in patients with renal disease. Thiazides decrease the glomerular filtration rate and increase azotemia.

Drug	Uses	Action	Dosage	Side effects	Nursing considerations
Hydrochloro-thiazide (Hydrodiuril, Esidrix, Oretic)	Mild-to-moderate heart failure; Hypertension	Same as chlorothiazide	*Oral only:* *Treat edema:* 25–200 mg/day in 1–3 doses; *Maintenance:* 25–100 mg/day; Onset: 2 hours; Peak: 4 hours; Duration: 6–12 hours	Hyperglycemia; Potassium depletion	Nursing considerations same as for chlorothiazide.
Triamterene, (Dyrenium), 50 mg plus hydrochloro-thiazide, 25 mg (Dyazide)	Edema; Mild-to-moderate hypertension	Blocks reabsorption of sodium in renal tubule; Interferes with exchange of sodium for potassium and H^+ ions	*Oral only:* 1–2 tablets/day; Onset: 1 hour; Peak: 2–3 hours; Duration: 7–9 hours	Hyperkalemia; Muscle cramps, weakness, dizziness, headache, and dry mouth	This drug conserves potassium and so is contraindicated in renal disease. Patients should not take potassium supplement.
Loop Diuretics (High-ceiling diuretics) Ethacrynic acid (Edecrin)	Edema of cardiac, hepatic or renal origin; Nephroses or chronic renal failure; Acute pulmonary edema (IV)	Inhibit sodium and chloride reabsorption in ascending loop of Henle; No direct acid-base change	*IV:* 50 mg and up; Onset: 5 minutes; *PO:* 50–200 mg/day; Onset: 30 minutes	Increased potassium excretion; Hyperuricemia and gout; Deafness	May potentiate ototoxic effects of other drugs

Table continued on following page

Table 17-7. DIURETICS (Continued)

DRUG	INDICATIONS	ACTIONS	USUAL DOSAGE	SIDE EFFECTS OR COMPLICATIONS	NURSING CONSIDERATIONS
Furosemide (Lasix)	Pulmonary edema (IV)	Same as ethacrynic acid	*Acute Use IV:* 20–200 mg	Electrolyte depletion	The oral form is used with Aldactone or Dyrenium to conserve potassium.
	Congestive heart failure		*Maintenance:* 20–80 mg/day PO	Potassium depletion can cause alkalosis	IV is used with aminophylline to potentiate diuresis.
	Given orally for mild-to-moderate hypertension		*IV Push:* Onset: 5 minutes	Dermatitis	If patient is refractory to previous doses, may be given as much as 1 gm per dose.
			Peak: 30 minutes	Tinnitus and hearing loss	
			Duration: 2 hours		Rapid, vigorous diuresis may increase blood viscosity and cause thrombi.
			IM: Peak: 1 hour		Patients with known hypersensitivity to sulfa may develop reactions.
			PO: Peak: 1–2 hours		
			Duration: 4–6 hours		
Potassium-sparing diuretics Triamterene (Dyrenium)	Mainly used in conjunction with other diuretics to reduce potassium loss	Increased excretion of sodium and chloride	*Oral only:* 100 mg 2 times/day	Side effects usually mild	Nausea can be reduced by giving the drug after meals.
		Maximum therapeutic effect occurs slowly	Peak: 1–2 hours	Nausea, vomiting, diarrhea	Hyperkalemia can result.
	Occasionally used for edema		Duration: 12–16 hours	Dizziness	Patients should not take a potassium supplement.
				Elevations of blood urea nitrogen (BUN), creatinine and chloride	

Table 17–8. VASODILATORS

DRUG	INDICATIONS	ACTIONS	USUAL DOSAGE	SIDE EFFECTS OR COMPLICATIONS	NURSING CONSIDERATIONS
Diazoxide (Hyperstat)	Hypertensive emergency	Arteriolar vasodilator	*IV:* Push: only 300 mg in 30 seconds	Severe hypotension to shock levels	This drug is ineffective in hypertension owing to pheochromocytoma.
			Peak: 1–5 minutes	Hyperglycemia	Patient should be supine when drug is given and remain so for 30 minutes after injection.
			Duration: 12 hours	CHF after repeated injections	
			Plasma half-life: 24 hours	Angina	Rapid injection (<30 seconds) allows for maximal therapeutic effects
				Arrhythmias	
				ECG changes	Patient requires close and frequent monitoring of blood pressure.
				Transient cerebral ischemia	
				Orthostatic hypotension	If this drug precipitates hypotensive crisis, give sympathomimetic agent such as norepinephrine.
				Flushing, sweating	
				Dizziness	Furosemide must also be given concurrently for maximum effect.
				GI discomfort	
				Pain along injected vein or at site of extravasation	

Table continued on following page

Table 17–8. VASODILATORS (Continued)

DRUG	INDICATIONS	ACTIONS	USUAL DOSAGE	SIDE EFFECTS OR COMPLICATIONS	NURSING CONSIDERATIONS
Erythrityl tetranitrate (Cardilate)	Relief and prevention of anginal attacks	Smooth muscle relaxer—especially finer blood vessels	*SL, CHEW, PO:* 10 mg ac and hs— may increase up to 100 mg/day Onset: SL and CHEW, 5 minutes; PO, 30 minutes Peak: SL and CHEW, 30–45 minutes; PO, 60–90 minutes Duration: SL and CHEW, 2 hours; PO, variable	Same as diazoxide	Known hypersensitivity is a contraindication to this drug.
Hydralazine hydrochloride (Apresoline)	Hypertension CHF	Arteriolar vasodilator ↓ Afterload	*IV:* Push: 20–40 mg in 20 ml at 1 ml/minute as necessary Drip: 50–100 mg/ liter IV fluid—titrate Onset: 10 minutes	Acute, reversible lupus syndrome Tachycardia Angina and associated ECG changes MI	When given by parenteral route, check blood pressure frequently. Watch for signs and symptoms of hypotension. This agent is contraindicated in patients with hypersensitivity to hydralazine.

Drug	Action	Use	Dosage	Adverse Effects	Comments
			IM: 10–60 mg as necessary; Onset: 30 minutes; Parenteral half life: 2–8 hours; *PO:* 10–50 mg q.i.d.; Peaks: 3–4 hours; Onset: 15–20 minutes	CHF; Postural hypotension; Tingling, numbness, paresthesia; GI disturbances; Headache, dizziness; Drug fever	Ingestion of alcohol may enhance adverse effects.
Isosorbide dinitrate (Isordil)	Smooth muscle relaxer	Relief and prevention of anginal attacks	*SL:* 2.5–10 mg q 2–3 hours; *CHEW:* 5–10 mg q 2–3 hours; *PO:* 5–60 mg q.i.d.	Headache, dizziness, flushing, weakness; Rash; Postural hypotension; Occasional severe hypotensive response, which may be seen even with low doses	
(Sorbitrate)	Same as isosorbide dinitrate	Same as isosorbide dinitrate	*SL and CHEW:* 2.5–10 mg prn or q 4–6 hours; Onset: 2–5 minutes	Same as isosorbide dinitrate	

Table continued on following page

SPECIFIC MEDICAL THERAPIES

314

Table 17–8. VASODILATORS (Continued)

DRUG	INDICATIONS	ACTIONS	USUAL DOSAGE	SIDE EFFECTS OR COMPLICATIONS	NURSING CONSIDERATIONS
(Sorbitrate) *Continued*			Duration: 1–2 hours		
			PO: 2.5–10 mg 3–4 times daily		
			Sustained action: 40 mg q 12 hours		
			Onset: 15–30 minutes		
			Duration: oral, 4–6 hours; sustained action, up to 12 hours		
Minoxidil (Loniten)	Severe symptomatic hypertension	Arteriolar vasodilator	*PO:* Initially 5 mg daily; may be increased up to 40 mg (max. dose 100 mg/day)	CHF	A diuretic and a beta-blocker or methyldopa should be used concomitantly.
	Severe hypertension proven refractory to usual maximum therapy		Plasma half-life: 4.2 hours	Tachycardia	Instruct patient about the importance of taking diuretics and a beta-blocker.
				ECG T-wave changes	
				Pericardial effusion and tamponade	

Drug	Action	Dosage	Side Effects	Nursing Considerations
Nitroglycerin (Nitrostat)	Smooth muscle relaxer; dilates smaller blood vessels, arterioles and capillaries Relief and management of angina Prophylaxis of angina attack prior to engaging in activities known to precipitate attack	SL or BUCCAL: 0.15 mg (1/400 gr) to 0.6 mg (1/100 gr) as needed Usual dose, 0.4 mg (1/150 gr) Onset: 2 minutes Peak: 5–8 minutes Duration: 15–30 minutes	Headache Dizziness Palpitations Reflex tachycardia Postural hypotension Syncope Too rapid blood pressure control, precipitating stroke or myocardial infarction (MI)	Encourage patient to report the following to the physician: Weight gain >5 lb (rapid) ↑ Heart rate (HR) >20 BPM ↑ Shortness of breath (SOB) Any new or more severe chest pain Severe indigestion Fainting or dizziness This drug is contraindicated in pheochromocytoma. As this agent may cause transient hypotension, lower head of bed (↓ HOB), keep patient supine and monitor closely until adequate blood pressure returns. *Patient teaching* guidelines are as follows: Tablets are light- and heat-sensitive; they should be replaced every 3 months to ensure potency. Sit down or lie down before taking They should have a "biting" or "tingling" quality in mouth if potent.

Table continued on following page

Table 17–8. VASODILATORS (Continued)

DRUG	INDICATIONS	ACTIONS	USUAL DOSAGE	SIDE EFFECTS OR COMPLICATIONS	NURSING CONSIDERATIONS
Nitroglycerin (Nitrostat) *Continued*					Patient may take up to 3 tablets, 5 minutes apart, for severe angina—if still unrelieved go directly to hospital emergency room (ER), preferably by aide vehicle. *Contraindications* Known hypersensitivity to nitroglycerin (NTG) ↑ Intracranial pressure Severe anemia
IV Nitroglycerin (Nitrostat IV)	Angina pectoris in patients unresponsive to organic nitrates and/or beta-blockers	Dilates venous and arteriole beds—venous effects predominate	*IV:* Bolus: 50 mcg every 3 to 5 minutes	Overdose: severe hypotension and reflex tachycardia	Nitroglycerin is absorbed by plastics—dilute and store in glass parenteral solution bottles only.
	Congestive heart failure associated with acute MI	Reduces both preload and afterload	Drip: Dilute 10 ml (8 mg nitroglycerin in 250 ml D_5W (= 30 mcg/ml)	Other: Headache, dizziness, cutaneous flushing	Use of special nonabsorbing infusion set is controversial.
	Perioperative: control of hypertension or production of hypotension		Average infusion via pump—5–20 mcg/minute	Tachycardia, bradycardia, nausea, vomiting, restlessness, muscle twitching	Continuous monitoring of BP, heart rate, and pulmonary artery wedge pressure (PAWP) is necessary to achieve correct dose.

2% nitroglycerin ointment (Nitrol Ointment, Nitro-Bid Ointment)	Treatment and prevention of anginal attacks	Same as nitroglycerin			*Overdose:* Since duration of drug-induced hemodynamic effects is usually quite short, elevation of patient's legs and decreasing or discontinuing the drug is often adequate treatment. Rarely, administration of an alpha-adrenergic agonist may be necessary (e.g., phenylephrine).
		May increase by increments of 5–10 mcg/minute every 3–5 minutes			
	Prevention of attacks of paroxysmal nocturnal dyspnea	Titrate to achieve desired hemodynamic effect—there is no fixed optimum dose	Headache, dizziness		Any convenient site of application is effective.
		Onset: 30 seconds	Postural hypotension		Remove old dose when applying new one.
		Topical:	Rash		
		½ inch to 5 inches q 3–6 hours (1 inch = 15 mg NTG)	Flushing		Teach patient how to use ruled tablet of paper to measure ointment and how to spread in a uniform layer on skin.
	Chronic treatment of left ventricular failure	Onset: 15 minutes	Weakness		
		Peak: 1–2 hours			If treatment is to be terminated, dosage and frequency should be gradually decreased over 4–6 weeks to avoid sudden withdrawal reactions.
		Duration: 3–4 hours			
					For contraindications, see under first nitroglycerin listings.

Table continued on following page

Table 17–8. VASODILATORS (Continued)

DRUG	INDICATIONS	ACTIONS	USUAL DOSAGE	SIDE EFFECTS OR COMPLICATIONS	NURSING CONSIDERATIONS
(Nitrodisc)	Same as for nitroglycerin	Same as for nitroglycerin	*Topical:* One disc per day Duration: 24 hours	Same as for nitroglycerin	
Nitroglycerin (Nitro-Bid plateau capsules)	Treatment and prevention of anginal attacks	Same as for nitroglycerin	*PO:* 2.5–9 mg q 8–12 hours	Same as for nitroglycerin	Alcohol enhances adverse effects. For contraindications, see under first nitroglycerin listing. The value of the use of long-action nitrates in treatment of angina is controversial.
Sodium nitroprusside (Nipride)	Hypertensive crisis Acute MI Acute left ventricular failure Refractory CHF	Potent peripheral vasodilator—acts directly on veins and arterioles—balanced effect Decreases both preload and afterload	*IV:* Drip only, per infusion pump Dilute, 50 mg in 500 ml D_5W (= 100 mcg/ml)	Profound hypotension Nausea and vomiting Dizziness, headache Chest pain, palpitations, reflex tachycardia	It is preferable to have arterial line. Keep patient supine. Be cautious with titration and monitoring of infusion.

| Aortic dissection with elevated blood pressure | Average dose: 0.5 to 8.0 mcg/kg/minute

Onset: 2–5 minutes

Duration: 5–15 minutes | Diaphoresis

Irritation at infusion site

Thiocyanate/cyanide toxicity (tinnitus, blurred vision, muscle spasms, psychosis, delirium) at doses >8 mcg/kg/minutes for >72 hours | Check blood pressure frequently and watch for signs and symptoms of hypotension/hypoperfusion.

Exposure to light causes deterioration—wrap IV bottle in foil or other opaque material.

Discard solution q 4 hours

If solution appears highly colored, discard; it should have faint brown tint.

It may be used in conjunction with dopamine drip to augment cardiac output.

If thiocyanate toxicity develops (blood level >10 mg/100 ml), stop drip and administer nitrites. |

Table 17–9. MISCELLANEOUS DRUGS

DRUG	INDICATIONS	ACTIONS	USUAL DOSAGE	SIDE EFFECTS	NURSING CONSIDERATIONS
Diazepam (Valium)	Symptomatic relief of anxiety and tension associated with acute MI	Induces calming effect by acting on parts of the limbic system, thalamus and hypothalamus	*IV:* Push: 2–10 mg as needed	Drowsiness	Do not mix or dilute IV Valium with other drugs or solutions.
	Prior to cardioversion to diminish patient's recall of procedure		Precardioversion: 5–20 mg IV, 5–10 minutes before procedure	Fatigue	Give IV push via slow injection.
				Impaired judgment and performance	Give IM deep injection.
			IM: 2–10 mg q 3–4 hours	Ataxia	Additive effects when taken with other CNS depressants such as alcohol.
	Anticonvulsant		*PO:* 2–10 mg 2–4 times daily	Apnea	When used with narcotic, may ↓ narcotic dose by one third.
					When using IV during precardioversion period, have resuscitation equipment, such as an Ambu bag, at hand.
Meperidine (Demerol)	Severe pain	*CNS:* Major action Analgesic Suppresses respiration	*IV:* Only route used for MI patients	Syncope associated with hypotension	Monitor vital signs during and after injection.
		Cardiovascular (CV): ↓ BP ↑ HR	25–100 mg, push slowly	Constipation and urinary retention (less common than with morphine sulfate)	Prevent postural hypotension.
		GI: Effects less than those produced by morphine	Effects peak in 1 hour and last for 2–4 hours	Tremors, muscle twitches, seizures, hyperactive reflexes	In bradycardia patients, it may be given in place of morphine.
					Use caution in patients with tachycardia, urinary retention and constipation.

Drug	Uses	Actions	Dosage	Side Effects	Nursing Considerations
Morphine sulfate	Severe pain. Dyspnea induced by left ventricular failure and pulmonary edema	CNS: Major action Analgesic. Alters psychologic response to pain. Suppresses anxiety and apprehension. Suppresses respiration. CV: ↓ Peripheral resistance and BP. ↓ Heart rate. GI: ↓ Motility	IV: Only route used for MI patients. 2–20 mg, push slowly. May give in 2- to 5-mg increments until pain is relieved. Effects peak in 20 minutes and last for 2½ to 6 hours	Respiratory depression. Nausea, vomiting and constipation. Hypotension and bradycardia. Increase intracranial pressure	Monitor respiration, BP and heart rate during and after injection. Prevent postural hypotension. Use caution in patients with bradycardia, chronic obstructive pulmonary disease, signs of urinary retention. This drug is contraindicated in patients with head injury. Prevent constipation by using a stool softener.
Potassium salts—in many commercial forms	Potassium deficiency induced by metabolic disorders (vomiting, diarrhea, and so on) and diuretics. Digitalis-induced arrhythmias	Decreases myocardial automaticity, excitability and conduction velocity	Depends on patient's requirement. IV: 20–100 mEq per day mixed with D_5W via continuous infusion; rate not to exceed 30 mEq/hour	Hyperkalemia, producing cardiac arrhythmias, heart block, decreased blood pressure, ECG changes ($\uparrow$ T and QRS, $\downarrow$ P), mental confusion, weakness of extremities, flaccid paralysis	Monitor cardiac rhythms, especially during high-dose IV infusion. IV infusion should be slow if possible to avoid discomfort in vein. A large vein should be chosen for concentration larger than 40 mEq/liter.

Table continued on following page

Table 17-9. MISCELLANEOUS DRUGS (Continued)

DRUG	INDICATIONS	ACTIONS	USUAL DOSAGE	SIDE EFFECTS	NURSING CONSIDERATIONS
Potassium salts—in many commercial forms *Continued*	Prophylaxis in patients with digitalis and diuretic therapy		*PO:* 20–100 mEq per day	Nausea, vomiting, diarrhea, abdominal discomfort	Oral potassium preparation usually is mixed with juice for better tolerance.
				Enteric-coated tablets may cause small bowel irritation and ulceration	Patient teaching may be needed for long-term compliance.
				Rapid IV infusion may cause bradycardia, heart block and sinus arrest	Dose should be lowered if patient uses salt substitute containing potassium.
					This drug is contraindicated in patients with renal disease and higher degree heart block (not induced by digitalis) and in those on potassium-sparing diuretics.
Sodium bicarbonate ($NaHCO_3$)	Metabolic acidosis	Buffers the acidotic state	*IV:* 1 amp (44 or 50 mEq) state; then 1 amp q 10 minutes as needed or until acidosis is corrected	Metabolic alkalosis	Arterial blood gases (ABGs) should be obtained for dose adjustment.
				CHF	Postarrest, watch for subsequent signs of pulmonary edema.
					Precipitation occurs in IV tubing if given simultaneously with $CaCl_2$.

SUGGESTED READINGS

Alpert, J. S., and Rippe, J. M.: *Manual of Cardiovascular Diagnosis and Therapy*, Boston, Little, Brown, 1980.

Dradup, K. A., et al.: The physiological basis for combined nitroprusside-dopamine therapy in post–myocardial infarction heart failure. *Heart and Lung*, 10:114, 1981.

Franciosa, J. A.: Nitroglycerin and nitrates in congestive heart failure. *Heart and Lung*, 9:873, 1980.

Frishman, W. H.: β-Adrenoceptor Antagonists: New Drugs and New Indications. N. Engl. J. Med., 305:500, 1981.

Gilman, A. G., Goodman, L. S., and Gilman, A.: *Goodman and Gilman's Pharmacological Basis of Therapeutics*, 6th ed. New York, Macmillan, 1980.

Loebl, S., Spratto, S., and Wit, A.: *The Nurse's Drug Handbook*. New York, John Wiley and Sons, 1977.

Melmon, K. L., and Morrelli, H. F.: *Clinical Pharmacology: Basic Principles in Therapeutics*, 2nd ed. New York, Macmillan, 1978.

Pepine, C. J., and Conti, C. R.: Caclium blockers in coronary heart disease. Parts I and II. *Mod. Concepts Cardiovascular Dis.*, 50:61, 1981.

Physicians' Desk Reference, 35th ed. Oradell, N.J., Medical Economics Company, 1981.

Ralston, S. E., and Hale, M. F.: *Review and Application of Clinical Pharmacology*. Philadelphia, J. B. Lippincott, 1977.

Rodman, M. J., and Smith, D. W.: *Pharmacology and Drug Therapy in Nursing*, 2nd ed. Philadelphia, J. B. Lippincott, 1979.

Schmidt, E., and Margolin, S.: *Harper's Handbook of Therapeutic Pharmacology*. Philadelphia, Harper and Row, 1981.

Ziesche, S., and Franciosa, J. A.: Clinical application of sodium nitroprusside. *Heart and Lung*, 6:99, 1977.

18

PACEMAKER

DEFINITION

A pacemaker is defined as a battery-operated generator that initiates and controls electrical stimulation of the heart via an electrode that is in direct contract with the myocardium.

TYPES

Temporary Pacing

The pulse generator is external, and the pacing electrode is inserted by transvenous or transthoracic route either at the bedside or under fluoroscopy. The electrode should be in direct contact with the endocardium. Its use is in emergent or temporary situations only (< 2 weeks). See Figure 18–1.

Permanent Pacing

The pulse generator is internal, and the pacing electrode is inserted in the operating room either by transvenous route

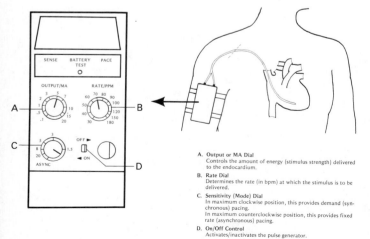

A. **Output or MA Dial**
Controls the amount of energy (stimulus strength) delivered to the endocardium.

B. **Rate Dial**
Determines the rate (in bpm) at which the stimulus is to be delivered.

C. **Sensitivity (Mode) Dial**
In maximum clockwise position, this provides demand (synchronous) pacing.
In maximum counterclockwise position, this provides fixed rate (asynchronous) pacing.

D. **On/Off Control**
Activates/inactivates the pulse generator.

Figure 18–1. Temporary pacemaker.

or directly applied to the epicardial surface by thoracotomy. Its use is in long-term management of symptomatic or life-threatening arrhythmias. See Figure 18–2.

Fixed Rate Pacing

At fixed rate pacing (asynchronous) (Fig. 18–3), the heart is stimulated at a continuous preset rate that is independent of its intrinsic electric activity. The disadvantage is that a competition between the paced beats and the patient's intrinsic rhythm may occur as a result of re-establishment of

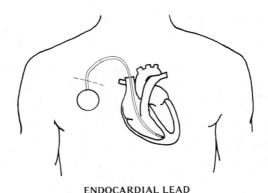

ENDOCARDIAL LEAD

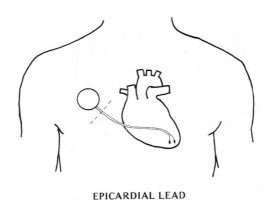

EPICARDIAL LEAD

Figure 18–2.   Permanent pacemaker.

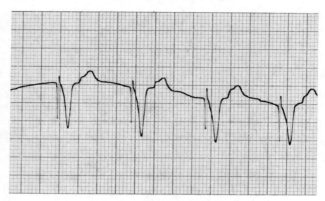

Figure 18–3. Paced rhythm.

atrioventricular (AV) conduction or appearance of ventricular extrasystoles. Consequently, it may lead to ventricular fibrillation. A fixed rate pacemaker is rarely used at the present time.

Noncompetitive Pacing

Noncompetitive pacing (synchronous) (Fig. 18–4) allows the heart to take over when AV conduction returns, rather than compete with it. There are two mechanisms:

Ventricular-Inhibited Type (Demand). The firing of the pacemaker is inhibited as long as the spontaneous ventricular rate is higher than the preset pacemaker rate. Pacing, therefore, takes place only when the ventricular rate falls below the preset level. In order for the pacemaker to sense the QRS, its amplitude has to be at least 0.5 mV (or depends on the manufacturer's specification). The disadvantage of this type is that the pacemaker may be falsely inhibited by tall T or P waves.

Ventricular-Activated Type (Standby). The firing of the pacemaker is triggered by each QRS and delivered immediately into it. If the spontaneous QRS complex fails to occur, the pacemaker will discharge at its preset delay interval. In order to prevent rapid cardiac stimulation or discharging upon

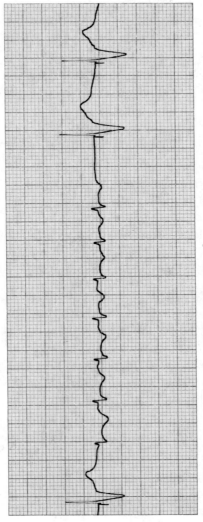

Figure 18-4. Synchronous pacing.

an early extrasystole, the pacemaker is designed with a refractory period of 0.4 second. Therefore, when the ventricular rate exceeds 150 per minute, the pacemaker is unable to sense or trigger the QRS. The disadvantages of this type are twofold:

a. When a premature beat appears too early to be sensed, the pacemaker may fire on the T wave of the premature beat.
b. The presence of a pacemaker spike in the normally conducted beats may alter the configuration of the QRS complexes.

Ventricular Pacing

The electrode is in direct contact with either the endocardial surface of the right ventricle or the epicardium of the left ventricle. Ventricular pacemakers may be temporary or permanent, fixed rate, demand or standby.

Atrial Pacing

The electrode is in direct contact with the atrium. Three mechanisms of atrial pacing are as follows:

Continuously Discharging. This type of pacemaker fires at a set rate. This mode can be used to terminate tachyarrhythmias by overdriving the tachycardia and recapturing the heart. The pacing rate is set higher than the arrhythmia rate. Once capture has been attained, the pacemaker is gradually decreased to a desired rate.

Demand. This kind of pacemaker is used when the sinus node fails but AV conduction is intact. This method maintains atrial contraction.

Synchronous. With this particular pacemaker, there are two electrodes: one in the atria and one in the ventricle. The atrial electrode senses the P wave and transmits the impulse to the ventricular electrode, which discharges after a suitable delay (A-V sequential pacing).

Unipolar Pacing

This pacemaker requires placement of a negative electrode within the heart and a positive electrode outside the heart (usually in the battery). Although unipolar electrodes are more sensitive to impulses within the heart and provide a more reliable "demand" function, their sensitivity to external interference increases the likelihood of false signals.

Bipolar Pacing

This type of pacemaker utilizes placement of both negative and positive electrodes in close proximity to the heart. The pacemaker spike is less prominent than that in unipolar pacing. Bipolar pacing is the most commonly used mode at present.

INDICATIONS

Pacemakers are generally indicated with symptomatic bradycardia, when the heart rate is insufficient to maintain an adequate cardiac output with resulting syncope, signs of heart failure or myocardial ischemia. It is also used for control (overdrive suppression) of refractory tachyarrhythmias. Specific indications are listed in Table 18–1.

COMPLICATIONS

These are summarized in Table 18–2.

NURSING IMPLICATIONS

During hospitalization for pacemaker insertion or manipulation, a defibrillator, emergency cart and appropriate medications should be available at all times for emergent use.

Table 18–1. INDICATIONS FOR PACEMAKER INSERTION

1. Asystole (emergency, temporary pacing)
2. Atrioventricular block
    a. Complete third-degree (Stokes-Adams, myocardial infarction)
    b. Second-degree (symptomatic or prophylactic)
3. Prophylaxis during cardiac surgery
4. Sick sinus syndrome
    a. Sinus arrest
    b. Sinus bradycardia (symptomatic)
    c. Bradycardia-tachycardia syndrome
5. Atrial fibrillation with slow ventricular response
6. Refractory tachyarrhythmia
    a. Sinus tachycardia
    b. Atrial tachycardia, fibrillation
    c. Junctional tachycardia
    d. Ventricular tachycardia

Table 18-2. COMPLICATIONS OF PACEMAKERS

COMPLICATION	CAUSE	CONSEQUENCES OF COMPLICATIONS
1. Failure to capture, pace, and sense (See Figures 18-5, 18-6, and 18-7)	Generator malfunction Break or loose connection anywhere in the system Manipulation or mishandling of generator or controls Runaway (>120 bpm); see Figure 18-8 Battery depletion Electromagnetic interference Catheter whip Displacement/misplacement of catheter in PA, neck, coronary sinus	Ventricular tachycardia (VT)/ventricular fibrillation (VF) Cardiac arrest Resumption of patient's inherent rhythm Demand mode reverts to fixed rate, resulting in competition with patient's spontaneous rhythm Diaphragmatic pacing
2. Infection of insertion site or pocket site	Casual sterility on insertion Poor wound care	Sepsis Loss of pacing
3. Electromicro shock (temporary pacemaker)	Exposed wires Contact with ungrounded equipment Wet external generator or wires	VF
4. Stimulation of diaphragm	Thin RV wall Ventricular perforation	Tamponade, hiccoughs at paced rate
5. Thrombophlebitis	Irritation in vein of entry	Obstruction to blood flow Embolization
6. Pneumothorax (temporary pacemaker)	Puncture of pleura during insertion	Respiratory distress Mediastinal shift
7. Fixed rate (asynchronous) competition with spontaneous rhythm	Return of spontaneous rhythm near or > set rate of pacemaker	VT/VF

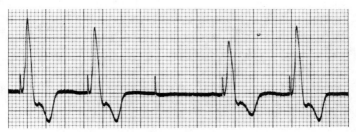

Figure 18–5. Failure to capture. (From Phillips, R. E., and Feeney, M. K.: *The Cardiac Rhythms*, 2nd ed. Philadelphia, W. B. Saunders, 1980, p. 347.)

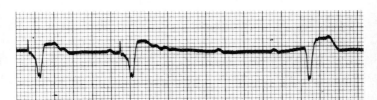

Figure 18–6. Failure to pace. (From Phillips, R. E., and Feeney, M. K.: *The Cardiac Rhythms*, 2nd ed. Philadelphia, W. B. Saunders, 1980, p. 346.)

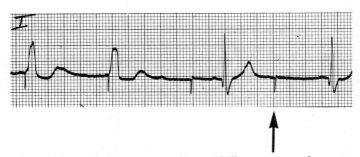

Figure 18–7. Failure to sense. (From Phillips, R. E., and Feeney, M. K.: *The Cardiac Rhythms*, 2nd ed. Philadelphia, W. B. Saunders, 1980, p. 358.)

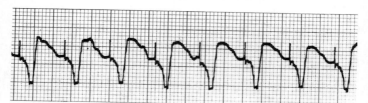

Figure 18–8. Runaway pacing rhythm. (From Phillips, R. E., and Feeney, M. K.: *The Cardiac Rhythms,* 2nd ed. Philadelphia, W. B. Saunders, 1980, p. 361.)

Temporary Pacemaker

Before Procedure

a. Explain to the patient and significant other the purpose (need) for a temporary pacemaker.

b. Allow the patient and significant other the opportunity to ventilate attitudes about pacemakers.

c. Have the patient sign the permission form for the procedure.

d. Gather the necessary equipment for the procedure (this will vary according to institution and chosen route of entry).

e. Check the functioning of the external generator (battery and sense and pace modes).

f. Check the patient's vital signs.

g. Obtain a rhythm strip.

During Procedure

a. Reassure the patient.

b. Monitor rhythm and vital signs.

c. Watch for and treat arrhythmia.

d. Determine and set stimulus and sensitivity thresholds and maintain setting per physician's instructions.

Stimulus Threshold. This should be 0.5 to 1.0 mA with a maintenance output of 5 mA (or 3 to 5 increments above threshold). If set too high, it results in irritability; if set too low, it results in failure to capture.

Sensitivity Threshold. This should be 6.0 mA (may vary owing to manufacturer's specifications) with maintenance sensitivity set in maximum clockwise position (unless oversensing is occurring). If set too high, it results in sensing of P or T as R wave; if set too low, it results in asynchronous pacing.

After Procedure
  a. Routinely check vital signs, temperature, heart rhythm.
  b. Tape or suture the electrode at insertion site.
  c. Secure all connections and routinely check connections as well as battery and control settings.
  d. Cleanse the incision with antiseptic solution; apply antibiotic ointment and sterile dressing. Label and date dressing. Change dressing daily or if wet.
  e. Keep the pulse generator dry and the controls protected from mishandling.
  f. Protect the patient from electromicro shock or electromagnetic interference.
      i. Cover exposed wires with rubber gloves or electrical tape.
      ii. Enclose the pulse generator in rubber glove (also keeps it dry).
      iii. Wear rubber gloves when handling exposed wires.
      iv. Avoid nurse-patient contact with electrical apparatus (e.g., unplug bed, do not use electric razor).
      v. Check for any ungrounded electrical equipment.
  g. If pacing or sensing malfunction occurs
      i. Secure all connections.
      ii. Check for proper control settings.
      iii. Check for battery depletion.
      iv. Reposition patient—turn to left side or change arm position.
      v. Try a different pulse generator (with same settings).
      vi. Notify physician (may need to increase mA or reposition catheter).
  h. Watch for diaphragmatic pacing (hiccoughs or diaphragmatic twitching at pacemaker's set rate).
  i. Encourage the patient and significant other to express feelings and fears regarding the pacemaker.
  j. Patient may be ambulatory if not contraindicated.

Permanent Pacemaker

Before Procedure
  a. A thorough explanation of the procedure should precede obtaining a signed consent. Usually only local anesthesia with mild sedation is used, as most permanent pacemakers are inserted via the transverse route instead of by epicardial implantation.

   b. Try to keep electrocardiographic (ECG) monitoring electrodes off the possible insertion site.

   c. Prep the area around the proposed insertion site, as dictated by hospital policy.

   d. A preoperative ECG should be obtained.

   e. The patient should be monitored in accordance with the underlying condition.

   f. A patent intravenous port should be maintained.

   g. Prophylactic antibiotics may be administered prior to procedure.

After Procedure

   a. Monitor vital signs at regular intervals.

   b. Check chest tubes if thoracotomy and epicardial implantation were done.

   c. Provide pain relief as needed. Often, oral analgesics provide adequate relief with transvenous insertion.

   d. Observe the operative site for inflammation and drainage.

   e. Monitor the patient for signs of pacemaker malfunction.

   f. Initially instruct the patient to avoid excessive extension or abduction of the arm on the operative site. Passive exercise may be performed to maintain range of motion in the joint.

   g. Obtain postoperative ECG, paced and nonpaced, if possible.

   h. Obtain postoperative posterior-anterior and lateral chest X-rays to check position of pacemaker electrodes.

   i. Encourage early ambulation. The patient may be up and about in the room on the same day.

   j. Record model and serial numbers of the pulse generator and leads. Include date of implantation and threshold measurements of initial implant.

   k. A pacemaker magnet may be used to test for adequate pacemaker function (by increasing and decreasing the set rate).

   l. Teaching of the patient is essential and should include the following:

      i. Inform the patient of the pacemaker set rate.

      ii. Have the patient take his or her own pulse daily for a full minute and report any slowing of heart rate or increase not associated with exercise.

     iii. Battery exhaustion is manifested by gradual slowing of heart rate by 5 to 10 beats over weeks.

(Present lithium and nuclear pulse generators have a life span of 5 to 20 years.)

iv. Report to the physician any of the following: vertigo, extreme fatigue, dyspnea, sudden weight gain, chest pain, swelling or drainage from incision and prolonged hiccoughs.

v. Caution the patient to avoid close contact with electrical appliances to avoid electromagentic interference and subsequent slowing of pulse. These appliances include microwave ovens, automobile engines, antitheft devices, electric razors, diathermy machines, television sets, and so on. It should be noted that this is less of a problem in appliances that are modern and in good condition.

vi. Stress the importance of regular visits to the physician.

vii. Encourage the patient to carry a pacemaker identification card.

m. Allow the patient to ventilate feelings regarding dependence upon the pacemaker and assure the patient that this should not significantly interfere with lifestyle.

SUGGESTED READINGS

Braunwald, E.: *Heart Disease*. Philadelphia, W. B. Saunders, 1980.

Furman, S.: Pacemaker emergencies. *Med. Clin. North Am.*, 63:113, 1979.

Mellar, S. (ed.): *Methods in Critical Care*. Philadelphia, W. B. Saunders, 1980.

Viebrock, R., and Barth, F.: The pacemaker patient: how you can spare him needless alarm. *RN*, 43:38, 1980.

19

CARDIOVERSION

DEFINITION

Cardioversion is the electrical reversion of a cardiac arrhythmia to normal sinus rhythm.

TYPE

Synchronous (Cardioversion)

The discharge of the electrical impulse from the cardioverter (or defibrillator) is synchronized with or triggered by the QRS complex of the patient's ECG. In most cases this type is used as an elective procedure.

Nonsynchronous (Defibrillation)

The discharge of the electrical impulse is not synchronized with the QRS complex. It is always used as an emergency procedure for ventricular fibrillation.

RATIONALE

When the self-sustained arrhythmia is momentarily abolished by an electrical shock across the chest wall, the entire myocardium is depolarized simultaneously and becomes refractory. The sinus node, with the highest intrinsic automaticity, will then have an opportunity to resume as the primary pacemaker.

INDICATIONS

1. Atrial flutter: often responds better to cardioversion than drug therapy.
2. Atrial fibrrillation: responds best to cardioversion when it has occurred less than 6 months.
3. Ventricular tachycardia accompanied by hypotension and pulmonary edema.

4. Supraventricular tachycardia causing hemodynamic embarrassment.
5. Ventricular fibrillation.

CONTRAINDICATIONS

Cardioversion should not be attempted in patients with the following conditions.

1. Longstanding atrial fibrillation.
2. Atrial fibrillation with slow ventricular rate.
3. Sick sinus syndrome with tachycardia and bradycardia combination.
4. Digitalis toxicity unless the rhythm is life-threatening.
5. Third-degree heart block.
6. Pre-existing conditions which prevent the patient from maintaining normal sinus.

GENERAL PROCEDURE

Cardioversion is performed by using a cardioverter (defibrillator), which consists of a capacitor discharge unit (direct current). The capacitor is capable of delivering shock up to 400 watt-seconds (joules), although the energy used may be as low as 10 watt-seconds. The electrical discharge is applied by using two insulated paddles placed on the chest wall along the long axis of the heart. The skin resistance should be reduced by using conductive paste, jelly or saline pads. The shock may be repeated with higher level of energy if the rhythm is not converted.

MEDICAL AND NURSING MANAGEMENT

Before Procedure

1. The procedure should be explained to the patient, and written consent should be obtained, unless the situation is a life-threatening emergency.
2. The patient should be NPO for several hours except for the prescribed oral antiarrhythmic drugs.
3. If the procedure is for atrial flutter or fibrillation, quinidine, 200 to 400 mg PO q 6 hours, is usually initiated 24 to 48 hours in advance to build up the serum level and

decrease the occurrence of postcardioversion arrhythmias.

4. The use of anticoagulants is still controversial. It usually begins several weeks prior to the procedure if it is chosen.
5. Preprocedure ECG and an intravenous line are required.
6. The potassium and digitalis levels should be within normal limits.
7. A crash cart with emergency drugs, oxygen, suction, and so on should be available.
8. The cardioverter should be turned on and switched to the synchronous mode and tested. For ventricular fibrillation, the synchronous mode *must not* be used.
9. Keep the room quiet and have the patient assume a comfortable supine position.
10. As a prophylactic measure, lidocaine bolus (50 to 100 mg) or other antifibrillation drugs may be given to the patient who has been on digitalis.
11. To produce an amnesic state, give diazepam in 5-mg increments IV (thiopental or barbiturates may be used instead) until the patient's speech is slowed.
12. Monitor and document vital signs.

During Procedure

1. Set the energy of the cardioverter at the selected level.
2. Prepare the skin by using conductive paste, jelly or saline pad.
3. Apply the paddles and deliver the shock.
4. Watch and record the change in cardiac rhythm.

After Procedure

1. Monitor and document vital signs and cardiac rhythms.
2. Twelve-lead ECG of newly converted rhythm is recommended.

COMPLICATIONS

1. Embolism, 1 to 2 per cent.
2. Ventricular ectopic beats, ventricular tachycardia and even ventricular fibrillation have been reported.

3. Myocardial injury may occur when multiple electrical discharges are delivered at high voltages of short intervals or when the paddle electrodes are small.
4. Hypotension.
5. Transient heart block.

SUGGESTED READINGS

Alpert, J. S., and Rippe, J. M.: *Manual of Cardiovascular Diagnosis and Therapy.* Boston, Little, Brown, 1980.
Braunwald, E.: *Heart Disease.* Philadelphia, W. B. Saunders, 1980.
Hurst, J. W., et al.: *The Heart, Arteries and Veins.* New York, McGraw-Hill, 1978.

20

CARDIOPULMONARY RESUSCITATION (CPR)

DEFINITION

Cardiopulmonary resuscitation (CPR) is defined as external maintenance of respiration and circulation during cardiac arrest by artificial ventilation and chest compressions.

INDICATIONS

Cardiac Arrest

Cardiac arrest is the abrupt cessation of circulation. Cardiac arrest occurs as a result of asystole, ventricular flutter or fibrillation, nonperfusing ventricular tachycardia or electro-mechanical dissociation (Table 20–1). It usually leads to respiratory arrest within seconds.

Respiratory Arrest

Respiratory arrest is the cessation of breathing. It may not cause cardiac arrest for several minutes.

GENERAL PROCEDURE

CPR is sequenced into categories of action according to priority, the ABCs (airway, breathing, circulation) of basic resuscitation and the DEFs (definitive therapy, emergent measures, follow-up) of advanced life support and management of cardiac arrest.

Airway

CPR begins with opening the airway by using the head tilt-chin lifting (or head tilt-neck lifting) maneuver. The head is tilted backward by pressing on the forehead while lifting the chin (Figs. 20–1 and 20–2). If cervical injury is suspected, the jaw thrust should be used. These maneuvers result in moving the tongue forward and sometimes will allow initiation of spontaneous respirations.

Table 20–1. INDICATIONS FOR CPR AND INTERVENTIONS IN PRIORITY ORDER

EVENT	INTERVENTION*
Asystole	CPR Epinephrine Atropine Sodium bicarbonate Calcium chloride or gluconate Pacemaker
Ventricular fibrillation or flutter	CPR Sodium bicarbonate Countershock, 200–300 watt-seconds (joules) Lidocaine bolus Epinephrine Bretylium
Ventricular tachycardia (nonperfusing)	Precordial thump CPR Countershock, 200–300 watt-seconds (joules) (synchronous) Sodium bicarbonate Lidocaine bolus Pronestyl 100 mgm IV Propranolol 1 mgm IV Bretylium
Electromechanical dissociation	CPR Calcium chloride or gluconate IV Epinephrine Sodium bicarbonate
Severe bradycardia, nontolerated	Atropine Supportive CPR Emergency pacemaker
Complete heart block, nontolerated	Atropine Supportive CPR Isoproterenol 1–8 mcg/minutes IV Emergency pacemaker

*See medication dosages in Table 20–2.

Breathing

Breathing or breathlessness is established by "look, listen and feel." The examiner places his or her cheek above the patient's mouth and nose while looking for chest movement and listening and feeling for air movement (Fig. 20–3). If breathing is absent, four "stacked" mouth-to-mouth breaths are given while pinching the patient's nose. The breaths are delivered rapidly to prevent previous breaths from fully escaping. The stacking should deliver from 800 to 2000 ml of air and re-expand collapsed alveoli.

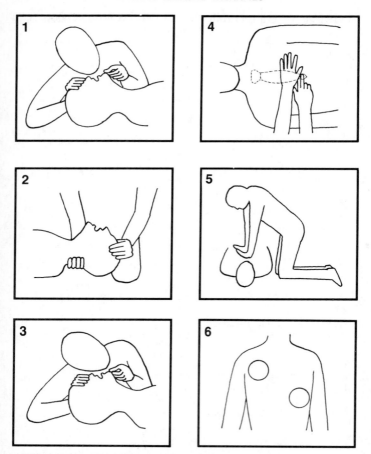

Figure 20–1. Head tilt-chin lifting.
Figure 20–2. Head tilt-neck lifting.
Figure 20–3. Establishing breathlessness by "look, listen and feel."
Figure 20–4. Hand position of chest compression.
Figure 20–5. Resuscitator's body position during chest compression—rocking forward until shoulders are directly over the patient's chest.
Figure 20–6. Position of defibrillator paddles.

Circulation

The carotid pulse is taken for 7 to 10 seconds. If the pulse is absent, chest compression is initiated. Sternal landmarks are noted by marking off two finger breadths above the sternal notch. The heel of one hand is placed in position above the two finger breadths with the other hand placed on top (Fig. 20–4). The fingers are extended or interlaced to prevent pressure on the chest wall. Chest compressions are accomplished by maintaining the elbows in a straight position with the shoulders directly over the patient's chest and rocking downward (Fig. 20–5). This method utilizes body weight rather than arm muscles and facilitates smooth, effortless compressions. A "50 per cent down, 50 per cent up" squeezing motion is more effective than the sharp, jerking motions that cause injury and are less effective in maintaining blood pressure. The hand position is lightly maintained between compressions to prevent position migration and fractured ribs. The sternum is depressed 1½ to 2 inches at a rate of 80 per minute. The femoral pulse should be monitored to assess the effectiveness of chest compressions. CPR should not be interrupted for more than 5 seconds. In one-person CPR, the ventilation and compression ratio is 2:15, and in two-person CPR, the ratio is 1:5.

Definitive Therapy

Therapy includes deliberate measures, defibrillation and drugs.

Adjunctive Airway Management. An *airway* should be inserted as soon as possible to maintain the tongue in a forward position. A ventilation bag should replace mouth-to-mouth resuscitation so that oxygenated air can be delivered.

Oxygen. One hundred per cent oxygen should be delivered as soon as possible.

Intravenous Lines. Heparin locks or keep-open intravenous lines are necessary for administration of drugs directly to the blood stream. Large-bore catheters are preferable, as they allow rapid injection of drugs. Two or more lines ensure access to the circulation and allow simultaneous injections of drugs or incompatible solutions.

Suction. Suction equipment should be available to maintain a patient airway and facilitate gastric decompression.

Defibrillation (Countershock). This is accomplished by discharging an electrical current through the heart and simultaneously depolarizing all of the cardiac cells, thus allowing a

Table 20–2. FIVE MOST COMMONLY USED RESUSCITATION DRUGS

DRUG	INDICATIONS	DOSAGE	LIMIT	NURSING CONSIDERATIONS
Sodium bicarbonate	Metabolic acidosis	1 mEq/kg initially, then 1 amp (50 mEq) q 10 minutes	3 amps until blood gases obtained	Excessive administration may result in alkalosis and/or sodium overload.
	Prior to countershock for ventricular fibrillation			Blood gases should be obtained as soon as possible to determine pH.
Epinephrine	Asystole	0.5 mg (5 ml of 1:10,000 solution); repeat at 5-minute intervals	—	Correct metabolic acidosis to enhance effect.
	Convert fine ventricular fibrillation to coarse ventricular fibrillation prior to countershock			If IV line is not available May give intracardiac. May instill in endotracheal tube.
				This drug is very short-acting, i.e., 5 minutes.
				Alkaline solutions destroy its effectiveness.

Drug	Indication	Dose	Maximum	Comments
Lidocaine	Ventricular tachycardia	50–100 mg q 3–5 minutes until arrhythmia suppressed	300 mg in 20- to 30-minute periods	Blood levels decline after 15–20 minutes. Seizures may result from doses greater than 300 mg. Continuous infusion, 2–4 mg/minute, should follow bolus.
Atropine	Bradycardia	0.5–1 mg q 5 minutes	2 mg	Atropine may cause ventricular tachycardia or ventricular fibrillation. Use with caution in digitalized patients.
Calcium chloride	Electromechanical dissociation / Asystole	2.5–5 ml of 10% solution or 250–500 mg *slow push* q 10 minutes	—	Rapid injection may cause severe bradycardia or sinus arrest. This drug precipitates if given with bicarbonate solutions.
Bretylium	Ventricular fibrillation and tachycardia	5–10 mg/kg/minute IV slow push; may repeat in 15–30 minutes; may be followed with IV drip of 1–2 mg/minute	30 mg/kg	Use with caution in digitalized patients. Severe hypotension may result or worsen if it already existed. IV push should be very slow.

single pacemaker the opportunity to take control. A conduction agent is first applied to the defibrillator paddles, or moist saline pads are placed in position on the chest. The paddles are placed on the chest wall along the long axis of the heart (Fig. 20–6). The paddles are pressed firmly against the chest wall to prevent leakage of current. The defibrillator is discharged at 200 to 300 watt-seconds (joules), depending on the size of the patient, the thickness of the chest wall and the rhythm being terminated. The paddle placement should be changed for repeated countershocks in order to avoid severe burning or blistering of the skin.

Drugs. Drugs are considered essential in cardiac resuscitation and are used to correct metabolic acidosis, to stimulate myocardial contraction, to accelerate cardiac rate and to suppress ventricular ectopy. The most commonly used drugs are listed in Table 20–2.

Emergent and Ancillary Measures

Emergent Measures. These measures include procedures that may be necessary to prolong life beyond the length of the code.

Intubation. Endotracheal intubation is the preferred method. Intubation facilitates suctioning and optimizes oxygenation.

Mechanical Ventilation. Ventilatory assistance is necessitated when respirations do not spontaneously return or the patient cannot tolerate the effort of breathing.

Pacemaker. Transthoracic or transvenous pacemakers may be indicated if asystole, severe bradycardia or complete heart block persists.

Vasopressor Agents. Hypotension frequently follows cardiac arrest and may continue to precipitate arrhythmias. Vasopressors commonly used are dopamine and norepinephrine.

Stomach Decompression. Severe abdominal distention can result from CPR and may compromise respirations. Nasogastric tubes relieve abdominal distention and prevent aspiration.

Ancillary Measures. These are measures that may not be directly related to saving the patient's life, but they should be attended to as soon as possible.

Documentation. An accurate ongoing record should be kept to document all procedures and medications given during the code. A flow sheet can be used as an immediate reference for the number of drugs given and should be kept as a permanent record of the event.

Reducing Overcrowding of the Environemnt.   Excess furniture should be removed from the area. Excess personnel can also interfere with access to the patient. It may be necessary to ask people to leave the room.

Provision of Information.   The patient's chart and the primary care giver who knows the patient or witnessed the precipitating event should remain at bedside to provide information to the resuscitation team.

Reassurance of Nearby Patients.   Patients within hearing and viewing distance of the code often are distressed by what they observe. They are usually aware of the gravity of the situation and, therefore, should be dealt with in an honest, reassuring manner.

Notification of Significant Others.   The patient's family should be notified of the critical nature of events. The nurse should also remember to notify all consultant physicians of the change in the patient's condition.

Follow-Up

Postresuscitation nursing care includes recognition of complications, diagnostic tests and close observation of vital signs.

Complications.   Those complications that may occur after CPR are as follows:

Trauma.   Improper chest compressions can cause fractured ribs, pneumothorax and ruptured spleen. Trauma injuries should especially be observed in patients who have been resuscitated by lay people. Pneumothorax is evidenced by respiratory distress, asymmetry of the chest or mediastinal shift. Ruptured spleen should be suspected in patients complaining of left upper quadrant pain and decreasing hematocrit.

Aspiration Pneumonia.   Cardiac arrest may precipitate vomiting in a semiconscious patient, creating a hazard for aspiration.

Anoxic Encephalopathy.   Brain death occurs at 4 to 6 minutes after unattended arrest. Prolonged hypoperfused states may leave the patient confused or exhibiting memory lapses.

Renal Failure.   Prolonged low-flow states may result in renal hypoxia and acute tubular necrosis (ATN). ATN begins 24 to 48 hours after renal hypoxia; the patient presents with decreasing urine output (less than 30 ml per hour) and increasing

BUN (greater than 20 ml/dl) and creatinine (greater than 1.5 mg/dl).

Heart Failure.　Overly vigorous use of sodium bicarbonate can cause sodium excess and result in heart failure. Increased heart and respiratory rate and pulmonary rales signal left ventricular failure.

Skin Burns.　Repeated defibrillation or delivery of high voltages can result in erythema and blistering of the skin.

Cardiac Tamponade.　Intracardiac injections or transthoracic pacemaker attempts incur the risk of perforation of cardiac structures and resultant extravasation of blood into the pericardial sac. Symptoms of tamponade include dyspnea, distended neck veins and narrowing pulse pressure.

Oral, Tracheal and Laryngeal Damage.　Emergency intubations and repeated intubation attempts may break teeth or cause soft tissue injury.

Cervical Neck Injuries.　Hyperextension of the neck during attempts to open the airway can result in cervical nerve trauma.

Diagnostic Tests.　These tests may detect complications and evaluate factors precipitating the arrest. Tests used are chest X-ray; electrocardiogram; laboratory studies, including CBC, arterial blood gases (ABGs), electrolytes and cardiac enzymes; and hemodynamic monitoring.

Vital Signs.　These should be taken every 15 minutes until the patient is stable.

Hourly Urine Measurements.　Urine should be measured until output exceeds 30 ml per hour for 6 to 8 hours.

Neurological Evaluation.　This should be done to assess cerebral hypoxia, if any. Orientation to time, person and place should be checked.

Psychological Support.　The patient surviving cardiac arrest may appear withdrawn and unwilling to verbalize or may converse obsessively by asking many questions. Regardless of the coping mechanism the patient chooses, anxiety is a predominant feature. The level of anxiety should be assessed to determine the need for therapeutic intervention. Appropriate information and assurance should be provided to the patient and the significant others, as indicated.

SUGGESTED READINGS

Budassi, S.: Management of cardiopulmonary arrest. *Nurs. Clin. North Am.*, 16:37, 1981.

Standards for Cardiopulmonary Resuscitation (CPR) and Emergency Cardiac Care (ECC). *J.A.M.A.*, 244:453, 1980.

Tyler, M. L.: Basic cardiopulmonary resuscitation. *Nurs. Clin. North Am.*, 13:499, 1978.

21

INTRA-AORTIC BALLOON PUMPING (IABP)

DEFINITION

Intra-aortic balloon pumping (IABP) is a method of providing circulatory assist to a failing left ventricle by a mechanical device (balloon pump) that utilizes the principles of counterpulsation. *Counterpulsation* means that the balloon inflates when the heart is in diastole and deflates when the heart is in systole.

RATIONALE

The two direct effects of counterpulsation are diastolic augmentation and afterload reduction.

Diastolic Augmentation

Diastolic augmentation results when the balloon inflates (pumps) during diastole and displaces blood, forcing it back into the aortic root. This results in an elevation of diastolic blood pressure, thus increasing coronary artery perfusion and oxygen supply to the myocardium.

Afterload Reduction

Afterload reduction results when the balloon deflates during systole, just before ventricular ejection. Deflation creates a forward blood flow, reducing resistance to left ventricular ejection and resulting in the following consequences: decreased ventricular wall tension during systole, decreased myocardial oxygen consumption, reduced ventricular size and lowered systolic blood pressure. Left ventricular output is improved, thus increasing cardiac output and decreasing venous congestion.

The net result of the two mechanisms is to increase oxygen supply and decrease oxygen demand, thereby reversing myocardial ischemia.

INDICATIONS

The balloon pump is used therapeutically and prophylactically to correct low-output states. The decision to use IABP should be made before prolonged deterioration reduces chances of survival.

Therapeutic Uses

1. Cardiogenic shock after acute myocardial infarction.
2. Cardiogenic shock after open heart surgery.
3. To assist weaning from cardiopulmonary bypass.
4. After acute myocardial infarction to limit infarct size (infarct containment).
5. Complicated myocardial infarction with severe heart failure or drug-resistant arrhythmias due to ischemia.
6. Unstable angina pectoris.

Prophylactic Uses

1. Before cardiac surgery to improve hemodynamic status.
2. During diagnostic procedure such as cardiac catheterization or arteriograms.
3. During noncardiac surgery on a cardiac patient.

CONTRAINDICATIONS

Selection of patients for IABP includes identifying those who will not be able to wean or those whose condition will be worsened by it. These include patients with severe aortic regurgitation, aortic dissection, old age, debility or terminal illness, pre-existing heart failure before recent infarct and abdominal aortic aneurysm or abdominoiliac, femoral graft.

GENERAL PROCEDURE

Insertion may be accomplished at the bedside, laboratory or operating room. The deflated, wrapped balloon, attached to a catheter, is inserted through a common femoral artery that has been stabilized with a graft or sheath. It is then quickly passed upward in the aorta until it lies in the descending aorta just distal to the left subclavian artery (Fig. 21–1). The catheter is connected to the gas-pumping apparatus (either helium or carbon dioxide is used) and to the control console, which also has an electrocardiogram input.

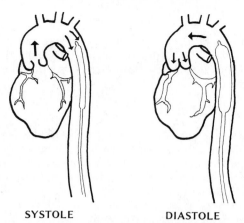

SYSTOLE DIASTOLE

Figure 21–1. Location of the intra-aortic balloon—in the descending aorta during systole and diastole.

COMPLICATIONS

1. Failure of the balloon to unwrap.
2. Malposition or migration.
3. Overinflation, resulting in intimal damage and hemolysis of red blood cells.
4. Underinflation, resulting in subtherapeutic effect.
5. Balloon rupture or leak.
6. Maltiming due to console failure.
   a. *early inflation*, leading to regurgitation into the left ventricle, or premature closing of the valve, thus increasing afterload.
   b. *Late inflation* into a particularly emptied aorta, decreasing augmentation and depriving coronary arteries of needed perfusion.
   c. *Prolonged deflation* lasting into the next systole and reducing unloading.
7. Aortic or femoral artery dissection.
8. Perforation of the common iliac artery during insertion.
9. Infection.
10. Emboli from the balloon, catheter or graft.
11. Limb ischemia of the cannulated limb, the most common complication.

MEDICAL AND NURSING MANAGEMENT

Before Procedure

1. Assessment of vasculature prior to insertion.
2. Insertion of an arterial line in upper extremities.
3. Prophylactic antibiotics.
4. Explanation of procedure to patient, including description of occasional "fluttering" patient may feel in the chest with inflation.
5. Signature of permit.
6. Preparation and shaving of groin.
7. Balloon size is selected from between 10 to 40 ml. The balloon should fill 85 per cent of the diameter of the aorta but not occlude it, as occlusion results in intimal damage and hemolysis of red blood cells. Aortic diameter is estimated from the size of the femoral artery and the patient's body surface area.

After Procedure

1. Timing.
   a. In *inflation*, the R wave of the ECG triggers the console to inflate for each heartbeat. The onset of inflation (augmentation) is adjusted to occur at the dicrotic notch of aortic wave form (Fig. 21–2), which indicates closure of the aortic valve.
   b. Deflation is adjusted to occur in the dip (Fig. 21–2) of aortic wave form, which represents the end of

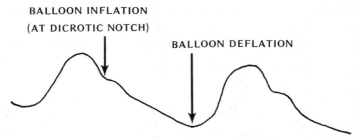

BALLOON INFLATION
(AT DICROTIC NOTCH)

BALLOON DEFLATION

Figure 21–2. Timing of balloon inflation at the dicrotic notch of aortic pressure wave form; balloon deflation at the dip of aortic pressure wave form.

diastole. The depth of the diastolic dip wave represents the amount of afterload reduction.

2. The catheter is frequently checked for kinks.

3. Hemodynamic monitoring is done to obtain cardiac outputs and to compute the filling pressures that result in the best cardiac outputs.

4. Laboratory studies include hematocrit and platelet counts, which monitor anemia and platelet destruction. Thrombocytopenia is common, with platelet counts often dropping below 100,000.

5. Chest X-ray should be done to check balloon positioning and symptoms of pulmonary edema or bleeding.

6. Positioning of the patient is done to relieve discomfort from all of the catheters and the inactivity they impose. The cannulated limb is prevented from flexing more than 30 degrees to avoid catheter movement.

7. Infection is monitored by frequent temperature checks, white blood cell (WBC) counts and inspection of the insertion site.

8. Hourly urine measurements are taken to monitor output.

9. Anticoagulation with heparin prevents thrombus occlusion of a limb.

10. Most important is frequent checks of peripheral perfusion of the cannulated limb for color, temperature and movement.

11. Psychlogical support should be optimistic, yet realistic. The shift to dependence on the IABP for maintenance of life often is done under urgent circumstances that accelerate the patient's anxiety. Frequent explanations of the equipment and the patient's condition should be offered.

12. For weaning, it must be kept in mind that the optimal effect of the pump is between 12 to 48 hours. Most patients are weanable by 5 days, with 10 days considered maximum. Requirements for weaning include the following:

    a. Patient is not taking vasoconstrictors and inotropic agents.

    b. Hemodynamic stability, including a mean arterial pressure greater than 60 mm Hg, a heart rate less than 110, a cardiac index greater than 2.1 and a filling pressure (PAWP) less than 20, stable or improving for 12 hours.

When the patient is deemed weanable, the pump is turned

off for 5 minutes. If there is no deterioration, cardiac assist is gradually decreased to a pumping:heartbeat ratio of 1:2 or 1:4 until it is no longer needed.

SUGGESTED READINGS

Boucher, M. J.: Intra-aortic balloon counterpulsation: current practices. *Crit. Care Q.*, 2:29, 1979.

Bregman, D.: Management of patients undergoing intra-aortic balloon pumping. *Heart and Lung*, 3:916, 1974.

Chrzanowski, A. L.: Intra-aortic balloon pumping: concepts and patient care. *Nurs. Clin. North Am.*, 13:513, 1978.

Whitman, G.: Intra-aortic balloon pumping and cardiac mechanics: a programmed lesson. *Heart and Lung*, 7:1034, 1978.

V

CARDIAC REHABILITATION

22

CARDIAC REHABILITATION OF THE MYOCARDIAL INFARCTION PATIENT

Cardiac rehabilitation includes teaching programs for patients with hypertension, angina, myocardial infarction, pacemakers and congestive heart failure.

This chapter describes rehabilitation and teaching after myocardial infarction. The teaching process for all cardiac conditions is the same, although the core content differs.

DEFINITION

Cardiac rehabilitation is the process of aiding an individual to adapt to the changes in lifestyle that result from a coronary event.

GOALS

The goals of cardiac rehabilitation change with the stages of adaption to the myocardial infarction.

Acute Stage

During the acute stage, the patient is often anxious and using denial. Goals are to reduce anxiety regarding hospitalization and to provide answers to the patient's question.

Intermediate Stage

In the intermediate stage, the patient has accepted the diagnosis, and formal education can begin. Goals are to inform the patient of factors contributing to the illness, to provide the patient with rationale underlying preventive health behavior and to aid psychosocial adjustment to the event.

Discharge Goals

Discharge goals are directed toward long-term outcome. They are to increase health behaviors, to maximize physical potential without endangering life and to reduce morbidity and mortality.

COMPONENTS OF CARDIAC REHABILITATION

Cardiac rehabilitation includes inpatient education, exercise prescription, psychosocial counseling and outpatient follow-up.

Patient Education

Knowledge is a coping skill that aids in the adjustment to an illness. Understanding of an illness is necessary if patients are expected to manage their lifestyles in healthful ways. Although a primary goal of patient education is to provide knowledge to the patient regarding the illness, the ultimate goal should be viewed in terms of the patient's outcome. Knowledge should be integrated with the patient's attitudes, beliefs and value systems in order to produce the desired behavioral outcomes.

Core Content.   Patients experiencing myocardial infarction have unique learning needs. They need to understand what caused the coronary event, how to manage pain or disability after the event and how to prevent reinfarction or complications in the future. The core content of post–myocardial infarction teaching programs addresses these needs.

Anatomy and Physiology.   This includes anatomy of the heart and pathogenesis of atherosclerosis and myocardial infarction. The healing stages of myocardial infarction can be related to the levels of activity restriction, thereby aiding the patient in understanding the importance of activity limitation.

Risk Factors.   Certain risk factors are highly correlated with coronary artery disease. The patient should be encouraged to identify his or her own risk factors and how they could be modified to reduce the potential for reinfarction. Modifiable risk factors include smoking, hypertension, obesity, diabetes, diets high in cholesterol and sodium, sedentary living and stress. When it is not realistic to attempt modification of several risk factors, those that impinge most heavily on future health should be emphasized.

Signs and Symptoms.   A major cause of death from myocardial infarction is delay in obtaining medical help. Patients should be able to recognize the signs and symptoms of a heart attack, or its complications, and know the appropriate action to take. They should also know the appropriate management of pain, dyspnea, palpitations and dizziness.

Medication Instruction.   The prescribing of any medication should include the name and dose of the medications, the purpose and effect of taking the medication, and any side effects or consequences from taking or not taking the medication.

Dietary Instruction. Any modification in diet should include explanation of the benefits of adherence to the diet and lists of foods that are recommended or to be avoided.

Activity Limitations. Once patients are not restricted by pain, they may have difficulty adhering to activity limitations. Activity restrictions should be clearly defined and posted in the patient's room (see Table 22–1).

Sexual Activity. Sex counseling includes when and how sexual activity can be resumed. Although many patients are reluctant to initiate discussion regarding their concerns in this area, they often need reassurance that sexual activity is safe.

The Process. The process includes the steps of assessment, planning, implementation and evaluation.

Assessment of Readiness to Learn. Before teaching begins, the patient should be physically and mentally ready for learning. This includes being mentally alert and free from pain and anxiety. Prior to this, only simple explanations should be offered. Readiness to learn is often signaled by the patient, usually by asking questions. When the patient is comfortable and indicates interest in or receptiveness to learning, formal teaching can begin.

Table 22–1. ACTIVITY LEVELS FOR PATIENTS IN THE CCU*

Level 0	Bedrest; passive range of motion to all major joints three times a day; assist with feeding and activities of daily living.
Level 1	May use commode, feed self and shave; dangle legs briefly with blood pressure and pulse recorded before and after activity twice a day
Level 2	Transfer to Intermediate Care area; chair, 30 minutes three times a day; record blood pressure and pulse with patient sitting and standing twice a day; change any TKO (to keep open) IV to heparin lock
Level 3	Chair, 45 minutes three times a day; may walk to the bathroom with assistance, with blood pressure and pulse recorded before and after once a day; may help with own bed bath; discontinue any IV that is TKO only
Level 4	Chair up to 1 hour four times a day; up in room as desired; shower or self-help bath permitted
Level 5	May walk length of hall three times a day, with blood pressure and pulse measured before and after, twice a day
Level 6	May walk as desired; may do own activities of daily living; blood pressure and pulse recorded before and after activity once a day

*Courtesy of Margaret Hall, M.D., Seattle, Washington.

Whom to Teach. Patients have the right to refuse education and not participate in teaching programs. They also should have the mental capacity to learn, an adequate attention span and physical ability to learn. Assessment also includes which family member or significant others should be involved in teaching.

Learning Needs. Learning needs are influenced by educational and ethnic backgrounds and by patients' value and belief systems. They are also dictated by the current concerns of the patient. For instance, it is not appropriate to pursue detailed descriptions of heart anatomy when the patient is preoccupied with job security or sexual ability.

Planning. The planning of patient teaching should be a cooperative process between patient and educator. Planning includes defining mutual objectives for outcome, selecting the teaching tools and projecting the time frame for completion of teaching.

Implementation. Patient teaching can be implemented by any one of, or a combination of, various methods.

Informal Teaching. Informal teaching is casual and unplanned. It constitutes a large part of the teaching of the patient, even within the context of a formal program. It allows for exchange of information between patient and instructor at times that may be more opportune for the patient. However, teaching that is done on a strictly informal basis is probably not as effective as planned teaching.

Formal Teaching. Formal teaching is organized and includes the following criteria: setting of learning objectives, documentation of teaching, and evidence that the patient has understood teaching.

Structured Teaching. This type of teaching follows specific, written guidelines that describe the content to be included and the time frame for completing each step of teaching. Written guidelines are useful in standardizing teaching among a group of instructors, and they help assist new nurses in knowing what and when to teach (see Table 22–2).

Individualized Teaching. Individualized teaching is done on a one-to-one basis and allows for participation of patients. The limitations and prognoses of patients are more closely considered, and teaching is tailored to fit individual needs.

Group Teaching. Group teaching is considered more cost effective because it requires less time to teach larger numbers of people. It also permits the members to share ideas and to learn from each other as well as from the instructor. However, individual needs often cannot be recognized in a group.

Table 22–2. CORONARY TEACHING GUIDELINES*

Acute Care: CCU
A. First day
   1. Obtain medical history.
   2. Explain to patient why he or she is in CCU.
   3. Assess patient and family psychosocial background, as well as readiness to take pretest.
   4. Pretest the patient, if condition permits, date and initial the test and record on chart.
   5. Explain the purpose of
      a. Monitor
      b. Oxygen
      c. IV
      d. Attendance of nurses
      e. Diagnostic tools, such as chest X-ray, ECG, blood tests
      f. General introduction to the CCU surroundings
   6. Teach patient to report chest pain promptly.
   7. Explain visiting restrictions.
   8. Instructions
      a. Visiting restrictions
      b. CCU routine
      c. Reporting of patient's condition
   9. Assess cultural, social, economic and educational background.
B. Second or third day
   1. Inform patient of diagnosis.
   2. Assess patient's interest in learning about and responding to diagnosis.
   3. Inform family of diagnosis.
   4. Assess family's response to diagnosis.
   5. Review psychosocial background.
   6. Discuss purpose of medications, when dispensed.
   7. Talk with patient about
      a. Definition of MI
      b. Definition and causes of angina
      c. Risk factors—controllable, including those that apply to patient
      d. Anatomy and physiology, including
         i. Circulation of blood through veins, heart, lungs and arteries
         ii. Coronary blood vessels
         iii. Plaque formation
         iv. Progression into heart attack
         v. Healing by scar formation
      e. Necessity of activity restrictions, including activity levels
   8. Document all information on patient's teaching record with date and initials; include individual's responses that may have an effect on teaching.

Transfer to Cardiac Rehabilitation Unit
A. Fourth day to discharge
   1. Orient to physical surroundings.
   2. Explain activity level.

Table continued on opposite page

Evaluation.   Evaluation of learning is an ongoing process. It is accomplished by measuring whether the objectives have been met and by observing behavioral changes. An effective means of measuring objective criteria is the use of pre- and post-tests. Pretesting is done before teaching is initiated and provides a baseline for knowledge assessment. Post-testing is

Table 22–2. CORONARY TEACHING GUIDELINES* (Continued)

Transfer to Cardiac Rehabilitation Unit (Continued)

    3. Inform family of different visiting privileges.

    4. Reassess interest for teaching.

    5. Present symptoms of heart attack, including those that patient may not have had.

    6. Tell patient about medications, including name, color, dose, purpose and frequency.

    7. Offer support systems, if necessary.

       a. Social services

       b. Clergy

       c. Community health agencies

       d. Nurse-psychologist

    8. Allow patient independence by

       a. Involvement in decision-making processes

       b. Taking part in personal hygiene routines

       c. Privacy whenever possible

       d. Reinvolvement with family structure

    9. Initial preparations for discharge

       a. Activity during first week at home

       b. Modification of lifestyle, to include

          i. Anxiety and depression

          ii. Return to work or routine activities of daily living

       c. Sexual activity

       d. Dietary consultation

       e. When to call a medic unit

       f. Complete scar formation—time element

Prior to Discharge

A. Duties of the nurse

    1. Post-test patient and record on documentation record.

    2. Arrange a 1-hour conference with family and patient to anticipate and answer questions about home care; discuss follow-up care with physician, medication and diet instructions, activity levels; and review and discuss test questions, clearing up any misconceptions or gaps in knowledge.

Discharge Packet

A. The packet should include the following items:

    1. Discharge instruction sheet from the hospital

    2. Medication information sheets with patient's own schedule of times and dosages

    3. Pamphlets and teaching aids relevant to home care and hospitalization

    4. Dietary information

    5. Medic II brochure

    6. Date for return to clinic for follow-up with physician

*Courtesy of Northwest Hospital, Seattle, Washington.

done upon completion of the teaching program; it documents learning and identifies areas that need further discussion. Meeting of behavioral objectives includes demonstration of manual skills such as pulse-taking or application of topical medications.

Documentation. Teaching should be documented either on a special record designed for this purpose (see Fig. 22–1) or

PATIENT TEACHING RECORD	Date:	Init.:	Comments:
I. Past Medical History:			
II. Orientation to Unit:			
III. Psychosocial Assessment:			

IV. Diagnosis: MI CHF Angina Hypertension Pacemaker			
V. Pretest: Date: Init.:			
VI. Controllable Risk Factors			
A.			
B.			
C.			
D.			

VII. Medications:	Comments:		Comments:
1.		4.	
2.		5.	
3.		6.	

VIII. Activity:

IX. Tools:

  A. Pamphlets

B. Teaching Tapes:	Date:	Init.:	
1. Heart Attack			
2. Risk Factors			
3. Intermediate Care			
4. Symptoms			
5. Going Home			
6. Sexual Activity			

C. Audiovisual:			
1. Myocardial Infarction			
2. Causes of Coronary Heart Disease			
3. Mr. Tense			
4. Hypertension			
5. Diet and Your Heart			
6. Coronary Heart Disease			

  D. Anatomy and Physiology

  E. Misc.

X. Diet:

XI. Post-test   Date: Init.:

XII. Conference and Evaluation: Date:

XIII. Take Home Packet:

  Comments:

Figure 22–1. Coronary patient teaching documentation.*

*Courtesy of Northwest Hospital, Seattle, Washington.

on a permanent part of the patient's chart. Documentation has two purposes: to communicate to each instructor where the patient is in the learning process and to record the learning accomplished.

Educational Resources.   Resources include both the teaching tools and the instructors.

Instructors.   Education of the patient, to some degree or other, is the responsibility of all members of the health team. However, nurses are in the optimum position to implement patient teaching and coordinate with other team members. Methods of organizing instruction are as follows.

Centralized Teaching.   In centralized teaching, a person or small core of persons such as clinical educational specialists are accountable for education of the patient. However, the main function of any centralized program should be to involve staff members in teaching, not to isolate them.

Decentralized Teaching.   This type of teaching utilizes nursing personnel equally, with each nurse assuming professional responsibility for teaching. This method is complementary to the roles of primary nursing.

Cardiac Rehabilitation Teams.   These offer the advantage of a multidisciplinary, holistic approach to education of the patient. The team can be assembled from nurses, cardiologists, dieticians, psychiatrists, psychologists, physical therapists, pharmacists, social workers and vocational therapists.

Teaching Tools

Written Materials.   These include pamphlets, many of which are available through national organizations such as the American Heart Association. Some teaching committees prefer writing their own materials in order to satisfy the goals of the program.

Audiovisual Aids.   These include audioteaching tapes or audiovisual cassettes that can be played at bedside. Closed-circuit television can be installed in hospitals for the purpose of educating patients.

Bedside Instruction.   Instruction is done on a one-to-one basis and allows for informal exchange of information and clarification of information the patient has received from other sources. Flip charts and heart models are useful for demonstration during bedside instruction.

Exercise Prescription

Activity is thought to enhance a feeling of return to normal and counteracts the effects of deconditioning after myocardial infarction. Low-level exercise testing can be completed before the patient is discharged in order to prescribe activity levels accurately for at-home activity. Treadmill testing of myocardial infarction patients should always be done under the supervision of a physician. The goal of prescription is maximum return to physical potential without threatening life or health. The exercise prescription is written in metabolic equivalents that are based on the results of treadmill testing. Patients are usually discharged with a prescription of 2 to 4 metabolic equivalents until the first office visit and are provided with a list of activities within the metabolic limitations (see Table 22–3).

Table 22–3. ENERGY COST OF VOCATIONAL AND RECREATIONAL ACTIVITIES*

METS†	VOCATIONAL	RECREATIONAL
2 or less	Desk work Driving cars, light trucks	Walk 1 mph, level Stitchery, needle crafts
2–3	Custodial work Typing, manual	Walk 2 mph, level Golf, riding cart
3–4	Mopping, hanging wash Driving trailer truck in traffic	Walk 2½ mph, level Golf, pulling cart
4–5	Interior carpentry Hoeing, raking leaves	Bicycle 8 mph, level Walk 3 mph
5–6	Light shoveling, digging General industrial labor	Walk 3½ mph, level Bicycle 10 mph
6–7	Splitting wood Shoveling snow	Walk 5 mph, level Bicycle 11 mph
7–8	Digging ditches Carrying 80 lb	Jog 5 mph, level Bicycle 12 mph
8–9	Tending furnace Moving van work	Run 5½ mph, level Handball and squash, social
10	Shoveling 10/min. 16 lbs.	Run 6 mph Handball and squash, competitive

*From Brammel, *H. L.* et al.: Physiological approach to cardiac rehabilitation. *Nurs. Clin. N. Am.*, 11:223–235, 1976.
†METS, metabolic equivalents.

Psychosocial Counseling

Nurses need to recognize when patients will benefit from psychosocial counseling. Such counseling may offer support in overcoming the natural anxiety and depression after a heart attack, may help with improving deficient coping skills, and may assist with occupational or personal adjustments. Spouses and significant others also may benefit from inclusion in the counseling.

Outpatient Follow-up

Despite having benefited from educational programs, patients often encounter problems after being discharged. They often do not know what they need to know until they return home and have to manage by themselves. Outpatient programs can help breach the gap between hospitalization and self-care. Postdischarge programs may include the following.

Postcoronary Group Classes.   In these classes, patients and families can share experiences and mutually resolve problems under the guidance of a medical professional.

CRP Classes.   CPR classes ensure that every patient's spouse, relative or significant other is trained in this technique after discharge of the patient.

Post–Myocardial Infarction Exercise Classes.   In these classes, patients go through graduated steps in exercise and reconditioning while under a physician's supervision.

SUGGESTED READINGS

Boggs, B., Malone, D., and McCulloch, C.: A coronary teaching program in a community hospital. Nurs. Clin. North Am., 13:457, 1979.

Brammel, H. L., and Niccoli, A.: A physiological approach to cardiac rehabilitation. Nurs. Clin. North Am., 11:223, 1976.

Dehn, M.: Rehabilitation of the cardiac patient: the effects of exercise. Am. J. Nurs., 80:435, 1980.

Johnston, B., Cantwell, J. D., and Fletcher, G.: Eight steps to in-patient cardiac rehabilitation. The team effort—methodology and preliminary results. Heart and Lung, 6:97, 1976.

McCulloch, C., Boggs, B., and Varner, C.: Implementation of educational programs for patients. Nurs. Admin. Q., 4:61, 1980.

Scalzi, C., Burke, L., and Greenland, S.: Evaluation of an in-patient education program for coronary patients and families. Heart and Lung, 9:846, 1980.

VI

APPENDICES

APPENDIX 1

FORMULAS AND PRINCIPLES

PRINCIPLES

Frank-Starling Law of the Heart

Within physiological limits, the greater the heart is filled during diastole (preload), the greater will be the quantity of blood pumped into the aorta.

Law of LaPlace

Wall (vascular or ventricular) tension is directly proportional to the pressure times the radius.

FORMULAS

Title	Formula	Normal Range
Cardiac output (CO)	= Heart rate (HR) × stroke volume (SV)	Stroke volume = 60–130 ml/beat
CO estimation by Fick principle	= $\dfrac{O_2 \text{ consumption}}{\text{AV } O_2 \text{ difference (ml/liter of blood)}}$	1–8 liters/minute
Cardiac index (CI)	= $\dfrac{CO}{\text{Body surface area (BSA)}}$	2.5–4 liters/minute/m^2
Ejection fraction (EF)	= $\dfrac{\text{Stroke volume}}{\text{End-diastolic volume}} \times 100$	67 ± 8
Pulse pressure	= Systolic pressure − Diastolic pressure	40–60 mm Hg
Mean arterial pressure (MAP) (average pressure throughout each cycle of heartbeat)	= Diastolic pressure + one third pulse pressure	70–100 mm Hg
Systemic (peripheral) vascular resistance (SVR)	= $\dfrac{\text{MAP} - \text{mean venous pressure}}{\text{CO (liter/minute)}}$	15–20 units
or	= $\dfrac{\text{MAP} - \text{mean venous pressure}}{\text{CO (liter/minute)}} \times 80$	900–1600 dynes/sec/cm^{-5}
Pressure rate product (PRP)	= $\dfrac{\text{Systolic BP} \times \text{HR}}{100}$	Compare with baseline value (at rest)

APPENDIX 2

SELECTED ANATOMY AND PHYSIOLOGY OF THE HEART

CORONARY ARTERIES

Left Main Coronary Artery

The left main coronary artery arises from aortic sinuses, is 1 to 2 cm in length and branches into the left anterior descending and left circumflex.

Left Anterior Descending. The left anterior descending (LAD) feeds the anterior interventricular septum, the anterior portion of the left ventricle and the whole apex.

Left Circumflex. The left circumflex feeds the posterior IV septum, the left atrium, the obtuse margin of the heart and its entire posterior wall.

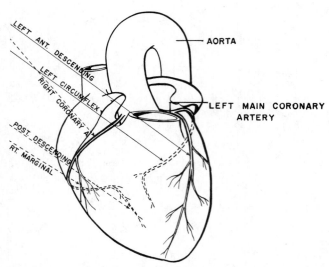

Figure A-1. Coronary arteries. (Modified from Rushmer, R.: *Cardiovascular Dynamics,* 4th ed. Philadelphia, W. B. Saunders, 1976, p. 363.)

Right Coronary Artery (RCA)

RCA feeds the posterosuperior IV septum, part of the left atrium, the right atrium, the SA node, the AV node, the right ventricle and the posterior and diaphragmatic walls of the left ventricle.

ACTION POTENTIAL OF THE VENTRICULAR MUSCLE CELLS AND PACEMAKER CELLS

Components of Action Potential

Phase 0
Depolarization of myocardium
Rapid influx of sodium ions into cell

Phase 1
First portion of cellular repolarization
Inactivation of sodium current

Phase 2
The plateau of repolarization
Shows influx of calcium ions into cell

Phase 3
Accelerated repolarization
Sodium and calcium expelled from cell
Potassium influx into cell

Phase 4
Membrane resting potential (MRP)
Inactivation of potassium current
In pacemaker cells, Phase 4 slowly rises owing to a gradual sodium influx (diastolic depolarization)
The degree of the slope of Phase 4 is one of the factors determining automaticity

Threshold Potential (TP). The TP is approximately -60 mV in atrial and ventricular muscle cells and -40 mV in the sinus node. This is a critical level at which the excitation of cardiac muscle takes place.

Absolute Refractory Period (ARP). The ARP includes Phases 0, 1, 2, and part of Phase 3. During this period, no stimulus can evoke an action potential.

Relative Refractory Period (RRP). RRP begins when the transmembrane potential in Phase 3 reaches the threshold potential and terminates just before Phase 3 ends. During

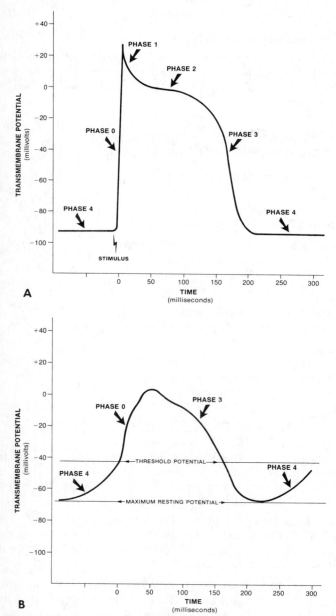

Figure A-2. *A*, Action potential of ventricular muscle cells. *B*, Action potential of cells in the sinus node. (From Phillips, R. E., and Feeney, M. K.: *The Cardiac Rhythms,* 2nd ed. Philadelphia, W. B. Saunders, 1980, pp. 16, 56.)

this period, only a strong stimulus can evoke an action potential.

Supernormal Period (SNP).   The SNP is a very brief period between RRP and the beginning of Phase 4.

Duration of Action Potential (DAP).   DAP includes the duration between the beginning of Phase 0 to the end of Phase 3. It represents systole.

Relationship Between Action Potential and ECG

Phase 0 = depolarization = QRS

Phase 1, 2, 3 = repolarization = ST − T $\Big\}$ = Systole
              These three phases are not distinguishable in pacemaker cells

Phase 4 = membrane resting potential = isoelectrical line
      = diastole

CONDUCTING SYSTEM OF THE HEART

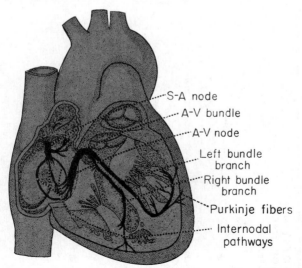

Figure A-3. Conducting system of the heart. (From Guyton, A. C.: *Textbook of Medical Physiology*, 6th ed. Philadelphia, W. B. Saunders, 1981, p. 165.)

DESCRIPTION OF THE CONDUCTING SYSTEM OF THE HEART

COMPONENTS OF CONDUCTING SYSTEM	DESCRIPTION	BLOOD SUPPLY	CONDUCTION RATE
SA node	Crescent strip (3 × 10 mm) in the posterior wall beneath and medial to the opening of superior vena cava. It is the pacemaker of the heart, with intrinsic rate of 60–100 beat/minute	SA node artery, 60–70% from RCA, 25% from LCA, 7% from both RCA & LCA	Rate in atria–1000 mm/second
AV node	On top of the intraventricular septum anterior to coronary sinus; it delays the transmission of impulses from atria to ventricles; intrinsic firing rate, 40–60/minute	80–90% from RCA, 10% from left circumflex artery	50 mm/second
Purkinje System	Including Bundle of His, bundle branches and Purkinje fibers		
Bundle of His	Connecting to the AV node	90% from RCA	
Bundle Branches	1. Right bundle branch is single small bundle of fibers 2. Left bundle branch is a large sheet of fiber and is divided into anterior/superior and posterior/inferior fascicles	Septal artery from LAD, except proximal few millimeters supplied by AV node artery	2000–3000 mm/second (Rate of ventricular myocardium: 200–500 mm/second)

CARDIAC CYCLE

Cardiac cycle represents the mechanical events of the heart during systole and diastole. The pressure changes, valvular openings and closures, and phonographic and electrocardiography happenings are illustrated in Figure A-4 and are briefly described in the following outline:

1. *Isometric contraction of the ventricles* (tension is increased in the muscle, but there is no shortening of muscle fibers).
   a. This begins shortly after the onset of QRS on ECG.
   b. AV valves are closed: S_1.
   c. Aortic and pulmonic valves are closed.
   d. The volume of blood in the ventricles is constant.
   e. Aortic pressure is about 80 mm Hg.
   f. The ventricular muscle fibers contract, but there is no blood flow (no emptying of the ventricles).
   g. Ventricular pressure rises steeply.
2. *Rapid ventricular ejection.*
   a. There is opening of aortic valve when left ventricular pressure > aortic pressure.
   b. There is rapid flow of blood from left ventricle to aorta.

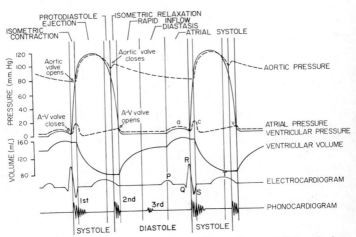

Figure A-4. Cardiac cycle and its relationship to ECG and phonocardiogram. (From Guyton, A. C. *Textbook of Medical Physiology*, 6th ed. Philadelphia, W. B. Saunders, 1981.

   c. Ventricular volume decreases sharply.

   d. Atria begin filling.

   e. Beginning of ventricular repolarization—beginning portion of "T."

3. *Decreased ventricular ejection (protodiastole).*

   a. The outflow rate of the ventricle decreases.

   b. Ventricular and aortic pressures begin to fall.

   c. Completion of ventricular repolarization is final portion of T.

4. *Isometric relaxation of ventricles.*

   a. Left ventricular pressure falls below the pressure in the aorta and pulmonary artery.

   b. Aortic and pulmonic valves are closed: S_2.

   c. Ventricular pressure continues to fall rapidly as ventricles relax.

   d. AV valves remain closed.

   e. Volume is constant in both ventricles.

   f. This period ends when ventricular pressure falls below pressure in atria.

5. *Rapid ventricular filling inflow* (the first third of diastole).

   a. AV valves are open when ventricular pressure < atrial pressure.

   b. Rapid ventricular filling begins.

   c. Aortic pressure slowly falls.

6. *Diastasis:* reduced ventricular filling (the middle third of diastole).

   a. Filling is less rapid.

   b. Filling is limited.

   c. Aortic pressure continues to fall.

   d. Volume and pressure in atria and ventricles are rising slightly.

   e. AV valves have long been open.

   f. Isoelectrical line on ECG.

   g. It is terminated by atrial contraction (the latter third of diastole).

7. *Atrial systole.*

   a. This occurs slightly after the beginning of the P wave.

   b. This slightly increases intra-atrial pressure.

   c. This slightly contributes to ventricular volume and pressure.

   d. Atrial relaxation follows ejection → then AV valves are closed.

   e. Pressure in the aorta continues to fall.

   f. S_4 may be heard.

   g. The ventricles begin to depolarize.

AUTONOMIC INNERVATION OF THE HEART

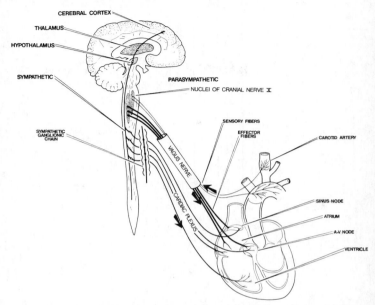

Figure A-5. Autonomic innervation of the heart. (From Phillips, R. E., and Feeney, M. K.: *The Cardiac Rhythms*, 2nd ed. Philadelphia, W. B. Saunders, 1980, p. 63.)

RELATIONSHIP OF HEIGHT AND WEIGHT TO BODY SURFACE AREA

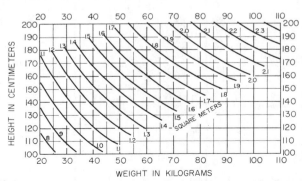

Figure A-6. Relationship of height and weight to body surface area. (From DuBois, E. F.: *Basal Metabolism in Health and Disease.* Philadelphia, Lea & Febiger, 1936.)

EFFECT OF AUTONOMIC NERVOUS SYSTEM ON THE HEART

TARGET AREA	PARASYMPATHETIC (Cholinergic, Vagus)	SYMPATHETIC (Norepinephrine)	ADRENERGIC Beta	ADRENERGIC Alpha
Sinus node	↓ Rate of firing	↑ Rate of firing	↑ Rate of firing	↑ Slight rate of firing
Atria	↓ Force of contraction	↑ Force of contraction	↑ Force of contraction	No effects
AV node	↓ Conduction speed	↑ Conduction speed	↑ Conduction speed	No effects
Ventricles	Little or no effects	↑ Force of contraction	↑ Force of contraction	No effects
Blood vessels	No effects	Vasoconstriction (dilation of coronary arteries)	Vasodilation (beta^2 effect)	Vasoconstriction

NOMOGRAM FOR ESTIMATING SERUM POTASSIUM CONCENTRATION

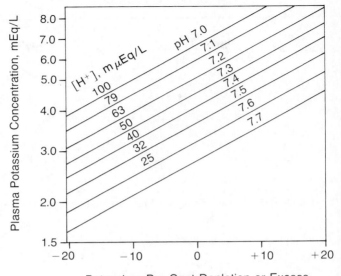

Figure A-7. Nomogram for estimating serum potassium concentration. (From Chapman, W. H., et al.: *The Urinary System: An Integrated Approach*. Philadelphia, W. B. Saunders, 1973.)

APPENDIX 3

PROCEDURE OF ADMITTING A PATIENT TO CCU

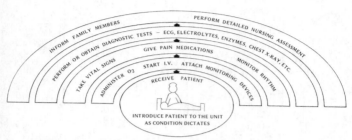

Figure A-8. Procedure of admitting a patient to CCU.

APPENDIX 4

CCU PHYSICIAN STANDING ORDER*

See pp. 383 to 385 for sample form.

*Courtesy of Northwest Hospital, Seattle WA.

Date —————

Check orders required.

ON ADMISSION

Admit CCU ——— ICU ——— 600's ———

Diagnosis ———————————

Activity ——————— Antiembolism hose ———

Monitor ——— Telemetry ——— Foot Board ———

500 c.c. D5W TKO (24 hours) ——— Heploc ———

Oxygen/prongs at ——— L/minute.

Oxygen prn chest pain ——— Oxygen/mask at ——— L/minute.

Diet ———————————

Salt substitute ———

EMERGENCY MEASURES

A. 1. Lidocaine 50–100 mg. I.V. bolus for PVC's greater than 6/minute.
    2. Lidocaine drip at 2 mg/minute after a 100 mg. lidocaine bolus for ventricular bigeminy, R on T, multifocal PVC's, ventricular tachycardia, or ventricular fibrillation. Lidocaine drip will consist of 2 gm. of lidocaine in 500 c.c. D5W.

B. In event of cardiac arrest:
    1. Defibrillation for ventricular fibrillation
    2. Sodium bicarbonate will be given *one* vial stat and *one every ten* minutes of arrest up to a total of *three* vials.
    3. Blood gases will be drawn.

C. Atropine ——— mg. I.V. for acute episode of pulse less than 40 beats/minute.

Appendix continued on following page

LABORATORY

Lab work and EKG's will be done during waking hours only unless the physician specifies another time.

CPK stat _____; in 12 hours _____; in 24 hours _____; in 36 hours _____

LDH stat _____; in 12 hours _____; in 24 hours _____; in 36 hours _____

Stat CBC _____ Urinalysis _____ Stat BUN _____ Stat blood sugar _____ Blood gases _____

Electrolytes stat _____; in 24 hours _____; in 36 hours _____

Chem profile _____ Other _____

EKG stat _____; in 24 hours _____; in 48 hours _____

Portable chest X-Ray _____ Other _____

MEDICATIONS

FOR PAIN
Nitroglycerin s/l 0.4 mg. prn pain _____.   Morphine 3–20 mg. I.V. prn pain _____.

Demerol 25–100 mg. I.V. prn pain _____.

FOR NAUSEA
Phenergan _____ mg. I.V. prn nausea.   Other _____

FOR SEDATION
Valium 5 mg. Q.I.D. _____.   Dalmane _____ mg. HS and MRxl

Other _____

LAXATIVES
Colace 100 mg. B.I.D. _____.   MOM 30 c.c. prn _____.

Other _____

                                        Signed _____ M.D./

Figure A-9. CCU Physician Standing Order. (Courtesy of Northwest Hospital, Seattle, Washington.)

ADMITTING NURSING CARE PLAN OF A PATIENT WITH MYOCARDIAL INFARCTION

A 40-year-old man was admitted to the Coronary Care Unit with complaints of substernal chest pain and "hyperventilation." He was initially very apprehensive and would tend to minimize his symptoms. Facial expressions of the patient indicated that he had more pain than he would admit. Only after repeated interviews did the patient finally admit the truth.

The patient stated that after his routine AM exercises (running in place) he experienced severe substernal aching, which radiated into his neck and left shoulder. Vertigo ensued, almost causing syncope. This frightened him. He also noted that his hands turned "numb" and felt extremely diaphoretic. He *denied* air hunger but noticed "hyperventilation."

HISTORY

Medical

This patient had no previous hospitalizations. He had been treated for several years for lupus erythematosus and had been experiencing intermittent finger stiffness and various joint pains. The patient also stated he had experienced several fleeting episodes of similar mild to moderate chest pain during the last year. These he attributed to his lupus and usually just took extra doses of prednisone. His only medication was prednisone, 10 mg t.i.d.

Social

1. Salesman for pharmaceutical company. Under recent job pressures. Finances adequate.
2. 6 ft 2 inches, 188 lb.
3. In process of divorce from wife of 17 years. This has caused him considerable anxiety and tension.
4. Three children ages 9 years to 16 years.

5. Activities include golf and tennis.
6. Hobbies: great fishing enthusiast; likes fly tying.

Risk Factors

1. No significant family predisposition.
2. Nonsmoker.
3. Under considerable pressure—primarily family difficulties.
4. Extremely anxious man. A definite Type A personality.

ADMITTING ASSESSMENT

Mental Behavior

The patient is alert and oriented, manifesting anxiety by talking continuously.

Cardiovascular System

The patient is complaining of severe 10/10 substernal crushing pain, radiating to the neck and left arm, requiring a total of 26 mg of morphine sulfate to obtain complete relief. Skin is pale, cool and clammy. The patient is afebrile. No neck vein distention or peripheral edema is noted. Blood pressure is 98/62 mm Hg bilaterally. Peripheral pulses are of normal quality and equal bilaterally. PMI is within normal limits (an instantaneous, single impulse at the fifth intercostal space in the midclavicular line). Auscultation reveals an S_1 greater than S_2 at the apex with an S_4 gallop present. Monitor shows sinus tachycardia, rate 104, with two short runs of ventricular tachycardia, necessitating a continuous lidocaine infusion at 3 mg per minute. Twelve-lead ECG reveals QS with elevated ST segments in V_1 through V_4.

Pulmonary System

Respiratory rate is 32/minute and shallow. Oxygen is administered per nasal prongs at 4 L/minute. Auscultation reveals bibasilar rales.

Gastrointestinal System

The patient has no complaints of nausea or vomiting. The abdomen is soft and nondistended with bowel tones present in all four quadrants.

NURSING CARE PLAN

PROBLEMS	GOALS	NURSING ORDERS	EVALUATION
1. Persistently recurrent chest pain, secondary to myocardial ischemia	1. Promptly and accurately report chest pain to nurse	1. Instruct patient about the importance of reporting and accurately describing pain (see pain protocol in Chapter 1)	1. Patient did not report pain unless asked
	2. Patient will acknowledge relief of pain	2. Promptly administer pain medication and document effect	2. Patient admitted relief following 26 mg morphine sulfate IV
		3. Identify precipitating factors and correlate with other symptoms	3. Pain occurred with no correlation to time or activity
2. Arrhythmias	1. Maintain HR < 90 at rest	1. Monitor changes in arrhythmias	1. Heart rate increased greater than 10 beats/minute after visit from estranged wife
a. Sinus tachycardia leading to increased myocardial workload		2. Correlative arrhythmia with time and activity	2. Strict bed rest enforced
b. Ventricular tachycardia; risk of ventricular fibrillation	2. Show no evidence of ventricular irritability	3. Minimize myocardial O_2 demand by bed rest, clear-liquid diet, sedatives, prompt pain relief, decreasing environmen-	3. Ventricular tachycardia requires lidocaine at 3 mg/minute to control

Nursing Diagnosis	Expected Outcomes	Nursing Interventions	Evaluation
3. Anxiety, secondary to pain and fear of death and potential impact on lifestyle	1. Patient will identify factors causing his anxiety 2. Subjectively, patient will acknowledge decrease in anxiety level	tal stimulation, stool softener and spacing nursing activity to allow for maximal period of rest 4. Give antiarrhythmic drugs as ordered and document effects and observe signs of toxicity 5. Assess tolerance to arrhythmia via vital signs, mentation and subjective complaints 1. Encourage and validate expression of feelings 2. Explore source of anxiety with patient and minimize controllable stressors 3. Maintain consistency in approach 4. Orient patient to CCU surroundings and nursing activities	4. No subjective symptoms of intolerance 1. Patient stated "I have done everything right. Why did this have to happen to me?" 2. "Does all this pain mean that I am going to die?"

Table continued on following page

NURSING CARE PLAN (Continued)

PROBLEMS	GOALS	NURSING ORDERS	EVALUATION
3. Anxiety, secondary to pain and fear of death and potential impact on lifestyle, *Continued*		5. Administer sedatives as ordered	
		6. Help patient to maintain control of his environment through decision-making when appropriate	
4. Early left ventricular failure, secondary acute myocardial ischemia	1. Decrease or absence of signs and symptoms of failure	1. Monitor for presence of or increase in rales, gallops, enlarged PMI, jugular vein distention, edema, ↑ respiratory rate and tachycardia	1. Persistent bibasilar rates and S_4
		2. ↑ Myocardial O_2 supply via O_2 administration (4 L/prongs)	2. Other parameters are within normal limits
		3. ↓ Myocardial O_2 demands as listed earlier under Problem 2	

APPENDIX 6

SELECTED MEDICATION TITRATION CHARTS—IN MICRODROPS
(1 ml = 60 gtt)

LIDOCAINE

Concentration = 2 gm lidocaine in 500 ml D_5W

Rate		Dosage
7.5 gtt/minute	=	0.5 mg/minute
15.0 gtt/minute	=	1.0 mg/minute
22.5 gtt/minute	=	1.5 mg/minute
30.0 gtt/minute	=	2.0 mg/minute
37.5 gtt/minute	=	2.5 mg/minute
45.0 gtt/minute	=	3.0 mg/minute
52.5 gtt/minute	=	3.5 mg/minute
60.0 gtt/minute	=	4.0 mg/minute

PROCAINAMIDE

Procainamide is administered as 2 gm in 500 ml D_5W. Rate and dosage are the same as for lidocaine.

BRETYLIUM

The concentration, rate and dosage are the same as for lidocaine and procainamide.

NITROPRUSSIDE (NIPRIDE) DOSAGE CHART

Concentration	=	50 mg/250 ml (200 mcg/ml)
Flow rate	=	microdrops/minute (gtt/minute)
Dosage unit	=	microgram/kg/minute (mcg/kg/minute)

lb / kg (gtt/min)	242/110	231/105	220/100	209/95	198/90	187/85	176/80	165/75	154/70	143/65	132/60	121/55	110/50	99/45	88/40	77/35
5	.152	.159	.167	.175	.185	.196	.208	.222	.238	.256	.278	.303	.333	.370	.417	.476
10	.303	.317	.333	.351	.370	.392	.416	.444	.476	.513	.555	.606	.667	.741	.833	.952
15	.455	.476	.500	.526	.556	.588	.625	.667	.714	.769	.833	.909	1.00	1.11	1.25	1.43
20	.606	.635	.667	.702	.741	.784	.833	.889	.952	1.03	1.11	1.21	1.33	1.48	1.67	1.90
25	.756	.794	.833	.877	.926	.980	1.04	1.11	1.19	1.28	1.39	1.52	1.67	1.85	2.08	2.38
30	.909	.952	1.00	1.05	1.11	1.18	1.25	1.33	1.43	1.54	1.67	1.82	2.00	2.22	2.50	2.86
35	1.06	1.11	1.17	1.23	1.30	1.37	1.46	1.56	1.67	1.79	1.94	2.12	2.33	2.59	2.92	3.33
40	1.21	1.27	1.33	1.40	1.48	1.57	1.67	1.78	1.90	2.05	2.22	2.42	2.67	2.96	3.33	3.81
45	1.36	1.43	1.50	1.58	1.67	1.76	1.88	2.00	2.14	2.31	2.50	2.73	3.00	3.33	3.75	4.29
50	1.52	1.59	1.67	1.75	1.85	1.96	2.08	2.22	2.38	2.56	2.78	3.03	3.33	3.70	4.17	4.76
55	1.67	1.75	1.83	1.93	2.04	2.16	2.29	2.44	2.62	2.82	3.06	3.33	3.67	4.07	4.58	5.24
60	1.82	1.90	2.00	2.11	2.22	2.35	2.59	2.67	2.86	3.08	3.33	3.64	4.00	4.44	5.00	5.71
65	1.97	2.06	2.17	2.28	2.41	2.55	2.71	2.89	3.10	3.33	3.61	3.94	4.33	4.81	5.42	6.19
70	2.12	2.22	2.33	2.46	2.59	2.75	2.92	3.11	3.33	3.59	3.89	4.24	4.67	5.19	5.83	6.67
75	2.27	2.38	2.50	2.63	2.78	2.94	3.12	3.33	3.57	3.85	4.17	4.55	5.00	5.56	6.25	7.14
80	2.42	2.54	2.67	2.81	2.96	3.14	3.33	3.56	3.81	4.10	4.44	4.85	5.33	5.92	6.67	7.62
85	2.58	2.70	2.83	2.98	3.15	3.33	3.54	3.78	4.05	4.36	4.72	5.15	5.67	6.30	7.08	8.10
90	2.73	2.86	3.00	3.16	3.33	3.53	3.75	4.00	4.29	4.62	5.00	5.45	6.00	6.67	7.50	8.57
95	2.88	3.02	3.17	3.33	3.52	3.73	3.96	4.22	4.52	4.87	5.28	5.76	6.33	7.04	7.92	9.05
100	3.03	3.17	3.33	3.51	3.70	3.92	4.17	4.44	4.76	5.13	5.56	6.06	6.67	7.41	8.33	9.52

Dosage: mcg/kg/min

Figure A-10. Titration chart for continuous intravenous administration of nitroprusside.

gtt/min \ Dosage	lb 77 / kg 35	88 / 40	99 / 45	110 / 50	121 / 55	132 / 60	143 / 65	154 / 70	165 / 75	176 / 80	187 / 85	198 / 90	209 / 95	220 / 100	231 / 105	242 / 110
5	3.8	3.4	2.9	2.6	2.4	2.2	2.0	1.9	1.8	1.6	1.55	1.5	1.4	1.3	1.25	1.2
10	7.6	6.7	5.9	5.3	4.9	4.5	4.1	3.8	3.6	3.3	3.1	3.0	2.8	2.7	2.5	2.4
15	11.4	10.0	8.9	8.0	7.3	6.6	6.1	5.7	5.3	5.0	4.7	4.4	4.2	4.0	3.8	3.6
20	15.2	13.3	11.8	10.7	9.7	8.9	8.2	7.6	7.1	6.7	6.3	5.9	5.6	5.3	5.1	4.9
25	19.0	16.6	14.8	13.4	12.1	11.1	10.2	9.5	8.9	8.4	7.8	7.4	7.0	6.6	6.3	6.0
30	22.9	20.0	17.8	16.0	14.6	13.3	12.3	11.4	10.7	10.0	9.4	8.9	8.4	8.0	7.6	7.3
35	26.6	23.3	20.7	18.6	17.0	15.5	14.3	13.3	12.4	11.6	11.0	10.3	9.8	9.3	8.9	8.5
40	30.5	26.7	23.7	21.3	19.4	17.8	16.4	15.2	14.2	13.3	12.6	11.9	11.2	10.7	10.2	9.7
45	34.3	30.0	26.6	24.0	21.8	20.0	18.4	17.1	16.0	15.0	14.1	13.3	12.6	12.0	11.4	10.9
50	38.1	33.3	29.6	26.7	24.2	22.2	20.5	19.0	17.8	16.7	15.7	14.8	14.0	13.3	12.7	12.1
55	41.9	36.6	32.6	29.3	26.6	24.4	22.5	20.9	19.5	18.3	17.2	16.3	15.4	14.6	13.9	13.3
60	45.7	40.0	35.6	32.0	29.1	26.7	24.6	22.9	21.3	20.0	18.8	17.8	16.8	16.0	15.2	14.6
70	53.3	46.7	41.5	37.3	34.0	31.1	28.7	26.7	24.9	23.3	22.0	20.7	19.6	18.7	17.8	17.0
80	60.9	53.3	47.4	42.7	38.8	35.6	32.8	30.5	28.4	26.7	25.1	23.7	22.5	21.3	20.3	19.4
90	68.6	60.0	53.3	48.0	43.6	40.0	36.9	34.3	32.0	30.0	28.2	26.7	25.3	24.0	22.9	21.8
100	76.2	66.7	59.3	53.3	48.5	44.5	41.0	38.1	35.6	33.3	31.4	29.6	28.1	26.7	25.4	24.3

Dosage: mcg/kg/min

Figure A-11. Titration chart for continuous intravenous administration of intropin.

INTROPIN (DOPAMINE) DOSAGE CHART

Concentration	=	800 mg/500 ml (1600 mcg/ml)
Flow rate	=	microdrops/min (gtt/min)
Dosage unit	=	microgram/kg/min (mcg/kg/min)

APPENDIX 7

ELECTRICAL SAFETY IN CCU

A continuous effort should be made to provide an electrically safe environment within CCU in order to prevent disasters such as shock, burn, arrhythmia, death, explosion, fire and power failure. Nurses should follow the safety precautions listed below:

1. Use a grounded outlet only. If necessary, attach all electrical equipment to a common ground wire, so leakage can be drained through a single pathway.
2. Unplug electrical beds if occupied by a patient with a temporary pacemaker.
3. Prevent a grounded patient from touching any device that might expose him or her to leakage of electrical current.
4. Prohibit the patient from using unauthorized electrical equipment.
5. Check the patient's cables for broken leads.
6. Check for open wires or broken plugs on the power cables leading to the patient or to staff-related equipment.
7. Report broken or discolored power outlets to plant operations.
8. Avoid using extension cords. If needed, used only 16-gauge/3-conductor wire with "NFPA"-approved hospital grade plugs on each end.
9. Test defibrillators for safe and accurate performance daily.
10. Report all calibration errors to biomedical service.
11. Have a biomedical service inspect monitoring equipment for current leakage, resistance and proper grounding once a month.
12. Have the plant operation's personnel check the operation of electrical beds every 6 months.

INDEX

Note: Page numbers in *italics* refer to illustrations; page numbers followed by (t) refer to tables.